ANATOMY OF
Yoga

THE MUSCLES IN YOGA

Blandine Calais-Germain

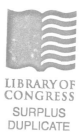

EASTLAND PRESS ❖ SEATTLE

Originally published as *Anatomie pour le yoga: Muscles et yoga*
Editions Desiris (France), 2017

English language edition © 2020 by Eastland Press, Inc.
P.O. Box 99749
Seattle, WA 98139, USA
www.eastlandpress.com

Library of Congress Control Number: 2019955454
ISBN: 978-0-939616-92-3

2   4   6   8   10   9   7   5   3   1

Printed in South Korea through Four Colour Print Group, Louisville, Kentucky

Translated from the French by Caitlin Barker
Book design by Gary Niemeier

Thank you to all the people who have collaborated
on the production of this book, in various ways:

Antonia Baumann
Bernard Bizeul
Matilde Cegarra
Éric Charrier
Bernard Coignard
Katia Cornier
Anne Debreilly
Sylvie Dugachard
Charlotte Fonseca
Romane Fossart de Rozeville
Jocelyne Galland
Gloria Gastaminza
François Germain
Nathalie Gérouard
Maria Gonzales
Elisabeth Jalabert
Ibai Lopez
Brigitte Masri
José Luis Marin Mateo
Hélène Mugica
Julia Roux

And thank you to the graphic artists
Marie-Luce Dehondt and Florence Penouty
for their enthusiasm…

Table of Contents

Foreword

. . . .

I practiced and taught dance, and training related to dance, for a long time. Then, having become a physiotherapist, I taught anatomy as it relates directly to movement (to understand it, and to put into practice that which knowledge of anatomy brings to movement).

This allowed me to meet practitioners and yoga teachers belonging to many schools over several decades. They came to lay down their mats in the Anatomy of Movement™ courses, and placed the skeleton molds on themselves to observe the vertebra in their own bodies, the position of the knee in Virasana, or the tripod of the foot, etc.

Gradually, content was created specifically for their needs: the teaching department AnatomYoga™ produces many theoretical contributions, analyses and practices of the poses, and preparatory training specific to certain poses. This content is still evolving, as the field of yoga is wide and varied.

Over the years, these courses have proven to be a fascinating laboratory of research and discovery, where knowledge passed down through the generations is discovered and reinforced.

In this context, I was often asked to write an anatomy book dedicated to yoga. The repertoire of poses being rather vast, I chose to limit it to one topic within the general subject, namely: "What happens to the muscles during yoga poses?" Their roles, in effect, are worth clearly distinguishing.

Thus this book is a journey through different muscle states, in order to inform the teaching and to renew the practice.

This book contains several types of content

It exposes the reader to many examples of asanas where the *muscles are brought into play* in various ways. The approach taken is to explore, through a detail of a pose, an aspect of the role of the muscles (sometimes found in a whole sequence).

- This takes the form of themed explanation sheets organized around a specific example such as a pose, a muscle, or a particular area in need of protection.
- Preceding or following these explanation sheets, you will find pages laying out theoretical concepts.
- Finally, some pages present lists of postures that are all associated with the same problem addressed in the explanation sheets.

Not everything that can be said about each pose is addressed. This is, rather, an occasion to observe an aspect of muscular behavior that might also be found in other poses. You don't have to read this book in a particular order: you can browse through the presentation of poses according to your own interests.

Note: This book is not a method for learning yoga. The poses are in no way presented in a progression (they do not, for example, progress from easy poses to more difficult ones). The level of difficulty of the poses observed has not been taken into account. The book is a tour of several situations where yoga is observed *in relation to the behavior of muscles.*

This book references the work *Anatomy of Movement*

The goal is not to describe basic human anatomy, but *to show how anatomy is implicated in the different asanas.* A little anatomy is brought in occasionally as it relates to the theme being discussed, and only as much as is necessary for understanding the theme.

For descriptions of basic anatomy, the book continuously refers the reader to pages in *Anatomy of Movement,* by the same author. This is indicated in the following manner: AOM, p. XX.

The "Themed Explanation Sheets"

Forty-three "explanation sheets" punctuate the reading. They aim to observe the muscles in yoga, *using real cases.*

Depending on the page, they present:

- the part played by *anatomy*
- situational *analysis*

- various hands-on *experiments*:
  - discovery of muscular action
  - lengthening of a muscle
  - palpation and identification
  - preparation for how to perform certain details of a pose
  - exercises for after a pose

How to use them:

Each explanation sheet is marked with a key. A label describes the nature of the content.

● ● ●   "PRACTICE AT THE END"

The content is first theoretical, and one or more exercises are introduced at the end of the explanation sheet.

● ● ●   "INTERMITTENT PRACTICE"

Theory and hands-on experiments are alternated throughout the explanation sheet.

◉   "SITUATION ANALYSIS"

The explanation sheet does not include examples or hands-on exercises, and should mainly be used to understand what happens to a muscle or what happens during a pose.

Abbreviations

The *vertebral column* will most often be called "the spine."

The *upper limbs* will often be called "the arms" and the *lower limbs* will often be called "the legs," as this is the common usage.

The *greater trochanter,* the massive bone projection at the top of the femurs, is often cited as it is the insertion point for many hip muscles. In the relevant pages, it is just called the "trochanter."

Flexion of the pelvis, extension of the pelvis are terms that describe movements of the pelvis that will be found on several pages. While standing with the pelvis flexed, the anterior superior iliac spines go both forward and downward. In extension of the pelvis, they go backward.

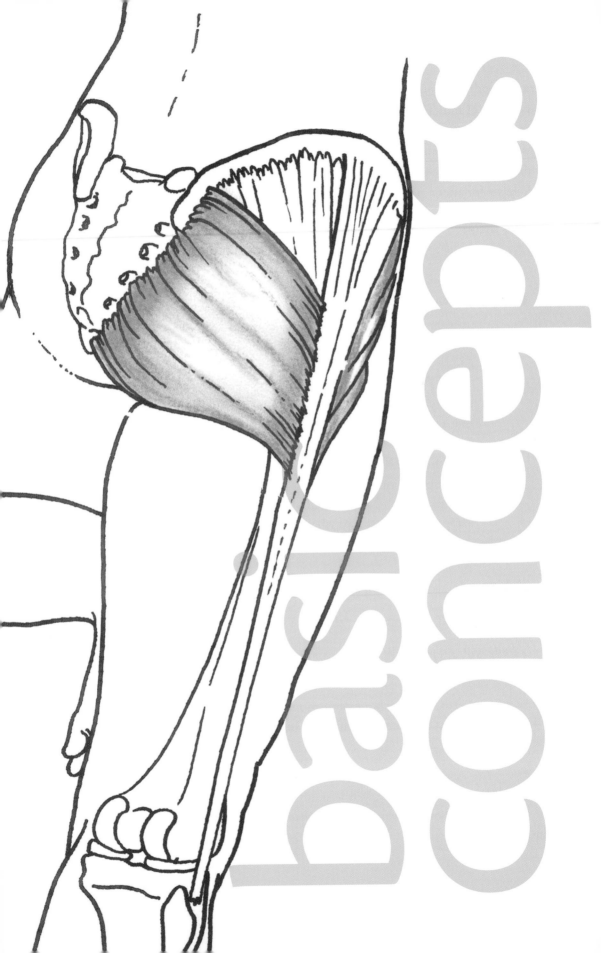

1

Some Basic Concepts About Muscles

These pages introduce some basic knowledge of muscles and their functions. It is not exhaustive, but presents what is necessary for understanding the rest of the book.

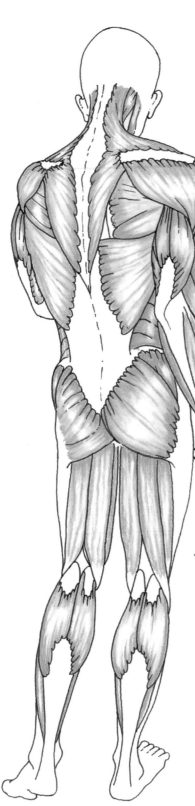

What is muscle?

Muscle is a kind of *tissue*. It is one of four types of tissue* that constitute the human body. A tissue is an arrangement of cells dedicated to a particular function in the body.

For muscles, this function is *contraction*.

The muscles discussed in this book

In the body there are three main types of muscles: cardiac muscle, smooth muscle (these two types do not concern us here), and skeletal muscles (also known as voluntary or striated muscles) which attach to and mobilize the skeleton.

It is only this last type of muscle that is observed here, in the context of certain yoga poses.

*Epithelial tissue, nervous tissue, connective tissue, and muscle tissue (to which a fifth type is sometimes added: blood tissue).

The structure of skeletal muscle, to the naked eye

Muscles are quite varied in *form* and *dimension*, but they all have one structure in common: when viewed in real size, you will see some *red* parts and some *white* parts.

The red parts are the only parts that can contract.

The white parts

> • either surround and divide the red mass
>   (these are the *aponeuroses*)

> or extend all the way to the bone
> (these are the *tendons)*

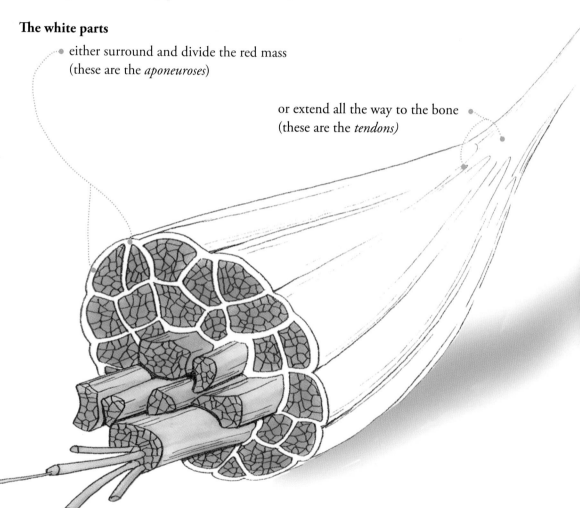

These white parts are *connective tissue*, which does not contract.

The structure of skeletal muscle, under the microscope

The red part is composed of supercells, called *muscular "fibers,"** which contain three kinds of proteins arranged within what are called *sarcomeres.*

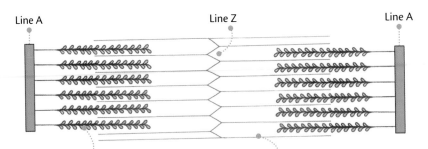

Line A   Line Z   Line A

Myosin proteins (in red), grouped into thick filaments (drawn in red), end with a curved "head" that plays a fundamental role in contraction. The filaments are connected at a transverse line: Line A.

Actin proteins (in blue), grouped into smaller-sized filaments, are inserted between the myosin filaments, and are connected to each other at a transverse line: Line Z.

Titin, a giant protein (the word comes from "titan"), connects Line Z to myosin and to Line A. It contributes to the maintenance and elasticity of the sarcomeres. It is presented on p. 100.

During muscle contraction, the actin and myosin filaments tend to get closer to one another and to commingle. A little like two hands "clasping their fingers together."

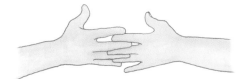

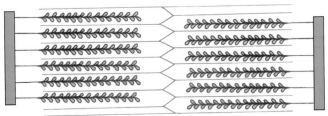

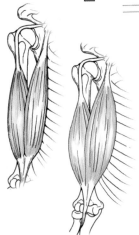

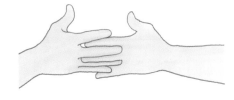

If this happens, the muscle fiber becomes shorter and thicker, as does the whole muscle on a larger scale. This shortening allows the muscle mass to pull the bones.

*The word "fiber" is commonly used instead of "cell" when discussing muscles, but it still refers to a cell.

When the muscle is stretched, these filaments tend to slide apart.

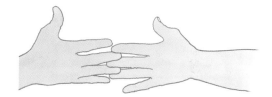

A little as if the same hands from before were releasing their clasp by sliding the fingers apart.

The arrangement of myosin and actin proteins forms a pattern that repeats throughout the length of the muscle fiber. A sarcomere is called the "basic unit" that goes from one Line Z to another. Just as a chain is composed of links, a muscle fiber is composed of sarcomeres.

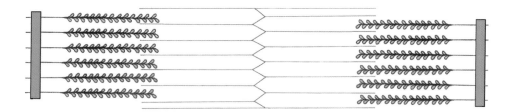

sarcomere   sarcomere   sarcomere

muscle fiber

It is this part of the muscle mass that responds to the reciprocal inhibition reflex (see p. 35).

The white parts are *connective tissue*, which consists of a fundamental substance in which cells and fibers are bathed, mainly collagen fibers and elastic fibers.

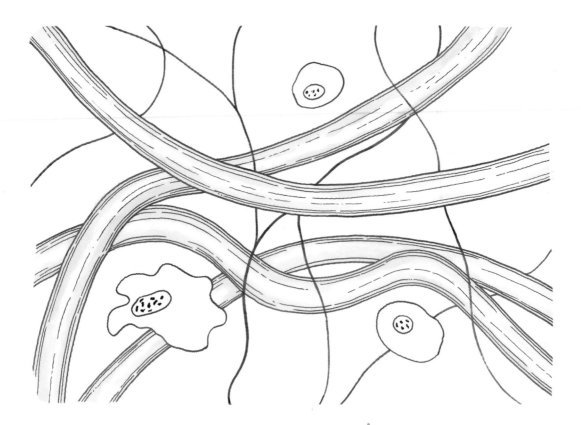

There are also other components, such as vessels and nerves, which are not shown in the drawing.

Connective tissue changes its name depending on where it is.

At the ends of the muscle, it takes the name *dense connective tissue*, to form *tendons*. It is resistant, and mostly retains its shape when faced with traction.

Around the mass muscle, it is called *areolar connective tissue,* and consists of a network of casings: the *aponeurosis*, which is divided in two so as to partition this mass increasingly finely. At the periphery of the muscle, this casing takes the name *epimysium*.

Deeper, it reinforces around the outside of packets of muscle fibers and is called *perimysium*, which is much thinner. Finally, it is divided again to encase each muscle fiber: this is the *endomysium*.

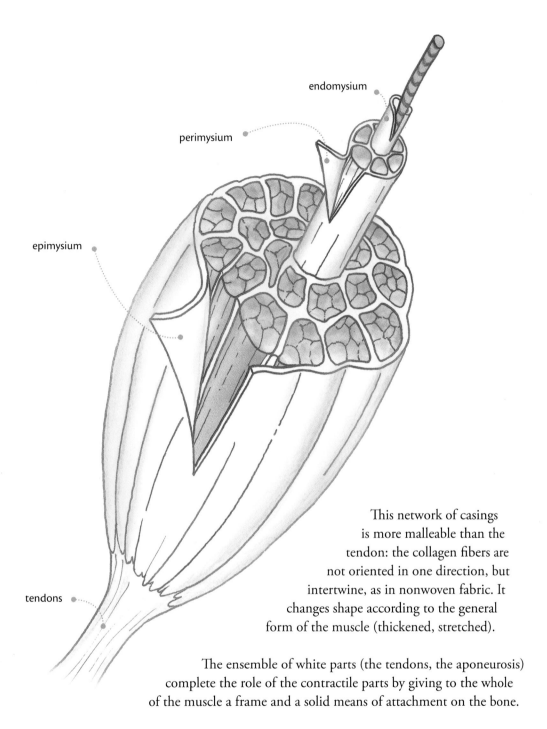

endomysium

perimysium

epimysium

tendons

This network of casings is more malleable than the tendon: the collagen fibers are not oriented in one direction, but intertwine, as in nonwoven fabric. It changes shape according to the general form of the muscle (thickened, stretched).

The ensemble of white parts (the tendons, the aponeurosis) complete the role of the contractile parts by giving to the whole of the muscle a frame and a solid means of attachment on the bone.

This part of the muscle mass does not respond to the reciprocal inhibition reflex (see p. 35), since this reflex rides on contraction/relaxation.

Muscles do not cause all movements

Muscular contraction creates a force that is the source of many movements, but not all: *many movements are caused by other forces.* In yoga, several actions are caused by *gravity.*

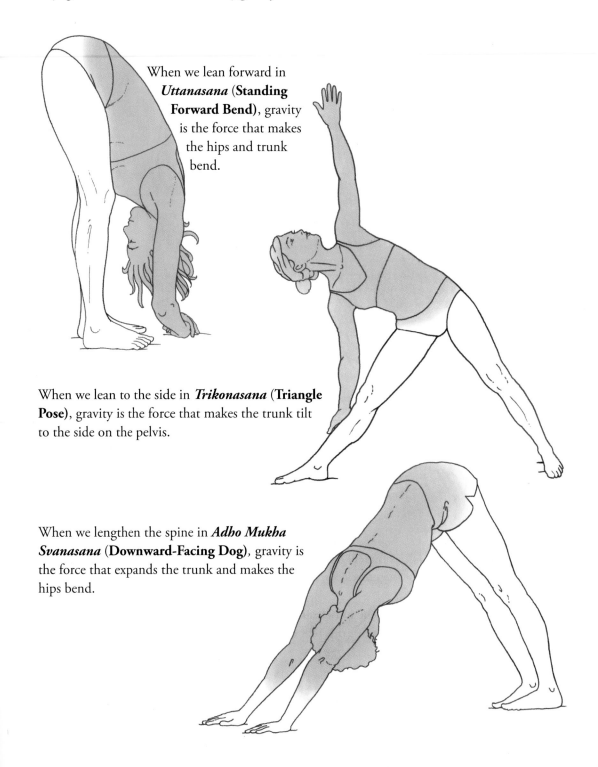

When we lean forward in ***Uttanasana* (Standing Forward Bend)**, gravity is the force that makes the hips and trunk bend.

When we lean to the side in ***Trikonasana* (Triangle Pose)**, gravity is the force that makes the trunk tilt to the side on the pelvis.

When we lengthen the spine in ***Adho Mukha Svanasana* (Downward-Facing Dog)**, gravity is the force that expands the trunk and makes the hips bend.

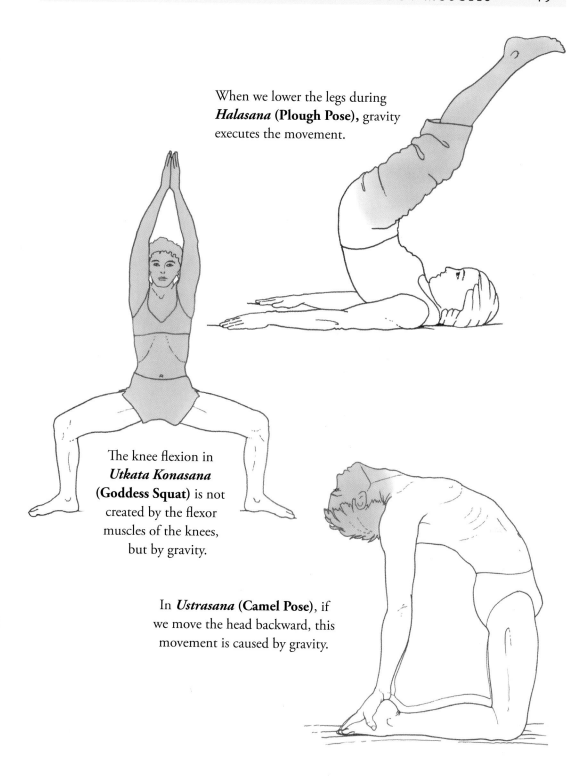

When we lower the legs during *Halasana* **(Plough Pose),** gravity executes the movement.

The knee flexion in *Utkata Konasana* **(Goddess Squat)** is not created by the flexor muscles of the knees, but by gravity.

In *Ustrasana* **(Camel Pose),** if we move the head backward, this movement is caused by gravity.

There are many other examples. Gravity is the actor in many movements or parts of movements. In these cases, muscular action combines with gravity to create the movement.

In the pose analyses in this book, this force will often be mentioned.

In addition to gravity, there are other forces at work in certain poses. Some examples:

When we claw the mat so as to pull and lengthen the trunk in *Marjarasana* (**Cat Pose**), the force is the supporting grip and traction.

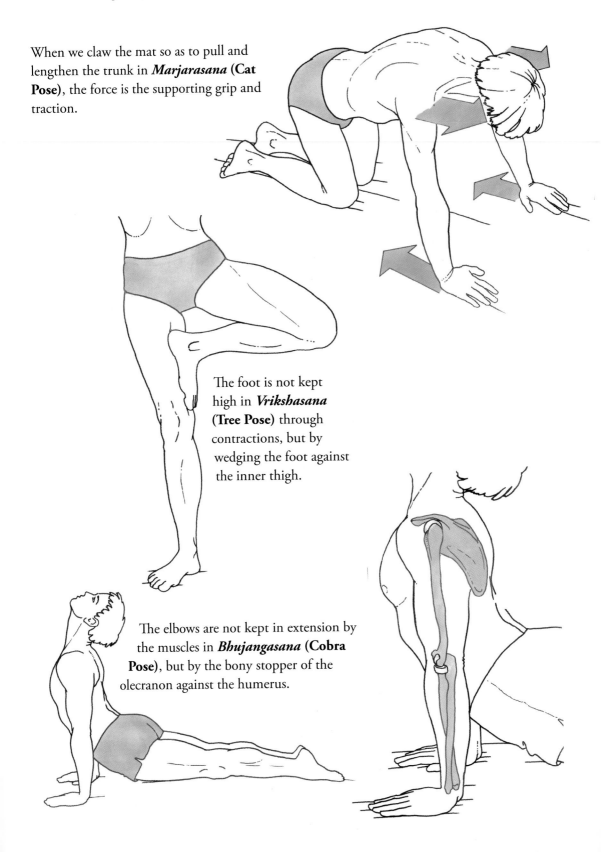

The foot is not kept high in *Vrikshasana* (**Tree Pose**) through contractions, but by wedging the foot against the inner thigh.

The elbows are not kept in extension by the muscles in *Bhujangasana* (**Cobra Pose**), but by the bony stopper of the olecranon against the humerus.

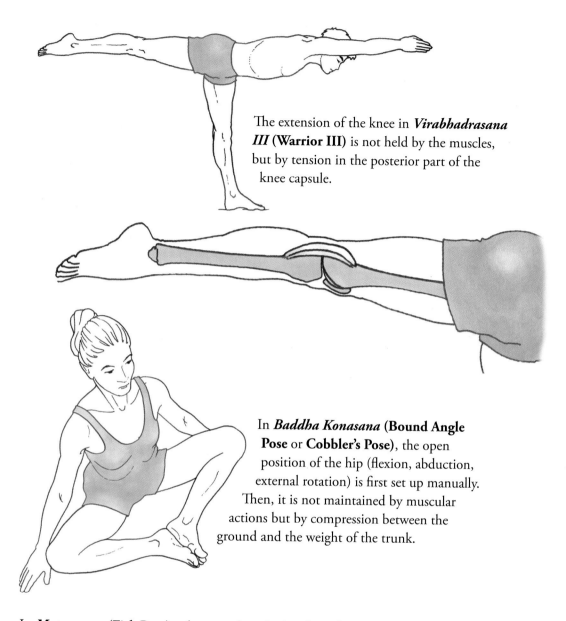

The extension of the knee in *Virabhadrasana III* (**Warrior III**) is not held by the muscles, but by tension in the posterior part of the knee capsule.

In *Baddha Konasana* (**Bound Angle Pose** or **Cobbler's Pose**), the open position of the hip (flexion, abduction, external rotation) is first set up manually. Then, it is not maintained by muscular actions but by compression between the ground and the weight of the trunk.

In *Matsyasana* (**Fish Pose**), when we place the hands under the buttocks, the hands are kept close together not through active muscle support, but due to the compression of the weight of the pelvis on the hands.

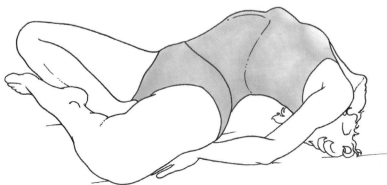

Muscles do not only act through contraction

A muscle can be a "passive tensor."

A heavily-stretched muscle turns into a traction rope. It no longer acts by being actively tightened, but rather like a tensed cable that pulls the bones without necessarily being contracted.

For example, in
**Paschimottanasana
(Seated Forward Bend),**
the movement of the pelvis
places the hamstring muscles
in tension. This in turn
frequently pulls the ischia
and pulls or keeps
the pelvis in
extension.

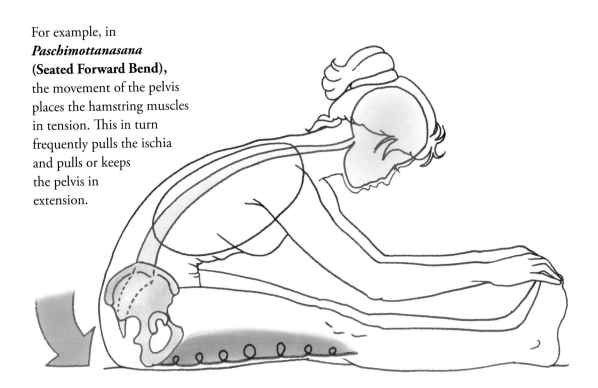

It is not the contraction of the hamstring
muscles that acts, but their *passive tension*.

This passive tension force is the result of having placed two structures in tension:

• unfolding and then placing the non-contractile white parts in tension (collagen fibers and the elastic fibers of the aponeuroses, see p. 16),

• unfolding and then placing in tension the titin proteins within the sarcomeres (see p. 16), which act as springs that resist stretching.

Agonist, antagonist, synergist...

For a given movement, the muscle that produces it is called the *agonist*.

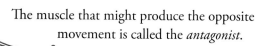

Example: the quadriceps, extensor muscles of the knee, are the agonist in an active extension of the knee.

The muscle that might produce the opposite movement is called the *antagonist*.

For example, the hamstring muscles, knee flexor muscles, are the antagonists of the quadriceps in an active extension of the knee.

When two muscles join together for a joint action, they are said to be *synergistic* for this action.

For example, the psoas, the sartorius, the tensor fasciae latae muscle, and the rectus femoris can act in synergy to flex the thigh on the pelvis.

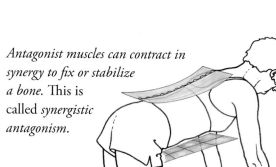

Antagonist muscles can contract in synergy to fix or stabilize a bone. This is called synergistic antagonism.

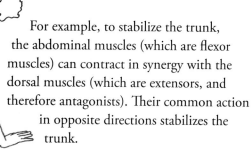

For example, to stabilize the trunk, the abdominal muscles (which are flexor muscles) can contract in synergy with the dorsal muscles (which are extensors, and therefore antagonists). Their common action in opposite directions stabilizes the trunk.

In poses, contraction takes different *forms*

During a pose, or when we move generally, the muscle can contribute to *producing* the movement.

For example, if the knee is extended in a seated position, when the foot rises above the ground, the action is *produced* by the contraction of the quadricep (which is, indeed, a knee extensor).

When a movement is made by an active muscle, we say that the contraction is *concentric*.

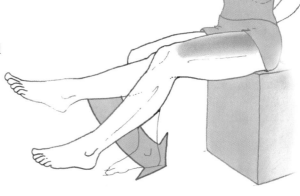

The same movement can then be performed in the other direction: we bend the knee, which makes the foot go back down. The force that pulls the leg and the foot is gravity. The same quadriceps muscle therefore works, not to produce the movement (which is produced by gravity), but to constrain the reverse movement, the bending.

When a movement is constrained by a muscle opposed to its action, we say that the contraction is *eccentric*. The muscle contracts while being lengthened.

These two forms of contraction have one thing in common: they are linked to movement, whether it is being produced or constrained. In yoga, they are put into play when entering and leaving the poses. This type of movement-related contraction is present in dynamic yoga forms like Ashtanga Yoga.

Even when there is no movement, muscles are
sometimes contracted. For example, if we *stay* a
moment at the end of the first movement, with the
knee straight: the quadriceps are still contracted.
But there is no movement.

This is called a stabilizing or
static contraction.

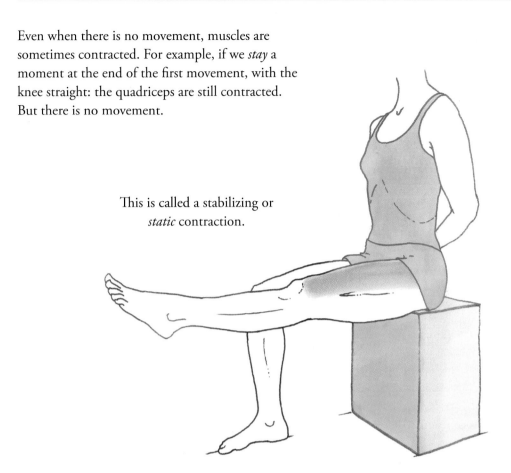

In yoga, once the pose is assumed we stay a certain amount of time *maintaining* it
(see p. 169).

At this stage, there is no movement (except for respiratory movements and small
adjustments). Maintaining this pose is, most often, a time of widespread static
contraction over the whole body.

In most schools of yoga, static contraction predominates.

Depending on the particular moment in the pose (beginning, maintenance,
conclusion), the same muscle will often alternate between concentric, static,
and eccentric contractions.

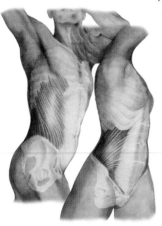

The same muscle can work *differently* depending on the pose

Here we will observe the case of the *external oblique* (and internal oblique), located on the side of the waist (AOM, p. 96). Their most posterior parts have fibers that go directly from the pelvis to the ribs. Their action brings the pelvis and the ribcage together, in lateral flexion. The obliques contract each time we shorten a side of the waist, but also each time that the waist is stabilized laterally, or when the opposite side of the waist is prevented from tilting.

Shorten one side of the waist

In order to do this, you can perform one of the ground variants of **Ardha Chandrasana (Half-Moon Pose)**.

First lie on one side of your trunk, arms above your head. Through a force that comes from the side of your waist, gradually curve the whole trunk, forming a crescent. Here, your obliques work very intensively, by shortening themselves on the side of your waist that faces up. The contraction is concentric.

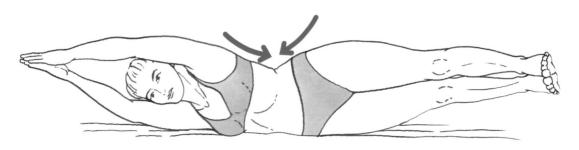

Stabilize the waist laterally

You can experiment with this by settling into the side variation of **Vasisthasana (Side-Plank Pose)**. Your obliques contract (but be careful: they are now working on the side facing down) to prevent your trunk from falling. They do not shorten, but just maintain the pose: their contraction is isometric.

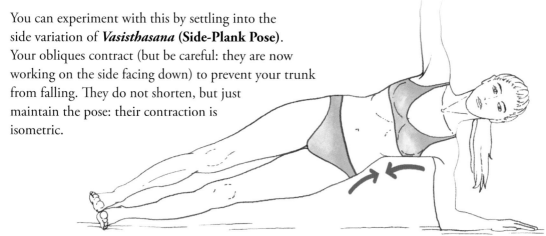

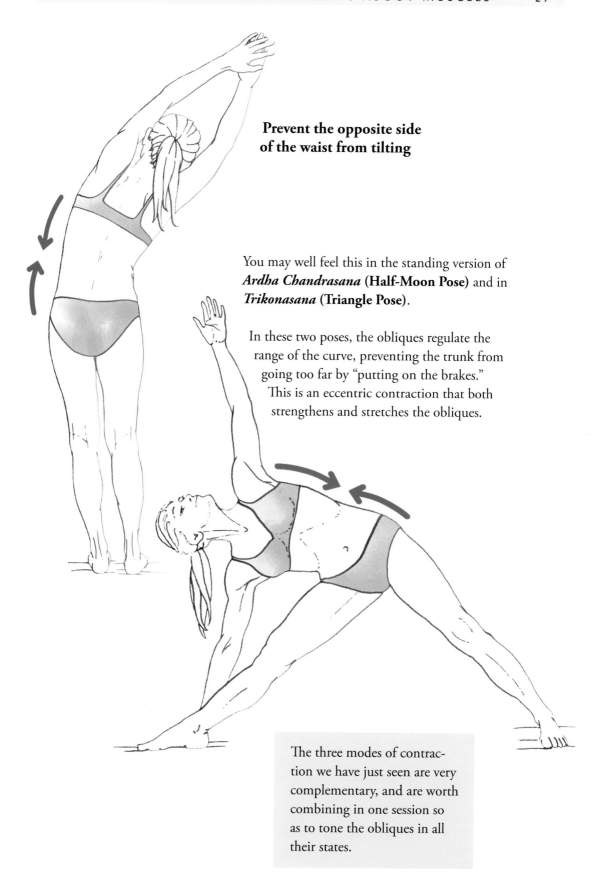

**Prevent the opposite side
of the waist from tilting**

You may well feel this in the standing version of
Ardha Chandrasana (Half-Moon Pose) and in
Trikonasana (Triangle Pose).

In these two poses, the obliques regulate the
range of the curve, preventing the trunk from
going too far by "putting on the brakes."
This is an eccentric contraction that both
strengthens and stretches the obliques.

The three modes of contraction we have just seen are very
complementary, and are worth
combining in one session so
as to tone the obliques in all
their states.

Contraction is not always where we imagine it to be

When we tilt the trunk in **Ardha Chandrasana** (**Half-Moon Pose**), the focalization goes to the side where the movement occurs. If we tilt to the right, we often think that the muscles are contracting on the action side.

But this is only true for a brief moment, at the very beginning of the movement: the muscles contract on the right in order to initiate the movement that puts the trunk out of balance towards the right. But immediately after, gravity takes over and strongly pulls the trunk so that it falls to the right.

It is then the muscles situated on the left side that contract, to restrain and slow the tilting. They work in eccentric contraction: they contract and are stretched at the same time.

In the curving or side-bending movements of the trunk from the vertical position, this pattern is very frequent: once past the (very brief) instant when the ipsilateral muscles initiate the movement, the muscular action is on the side opposite the direction of curvature, so as to hold it.

It is important to think in the right way about this, since the action protects the disks and nerves, and should not be forgotten.

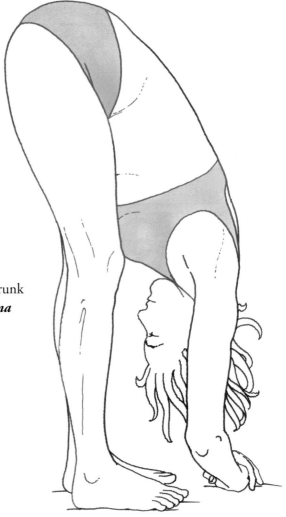

This is found in poses where the trunk bends forward: **Paschimottanasana** (**Seated Forward-Bend**) and **Uttanasana** (**Forward Bend**)...

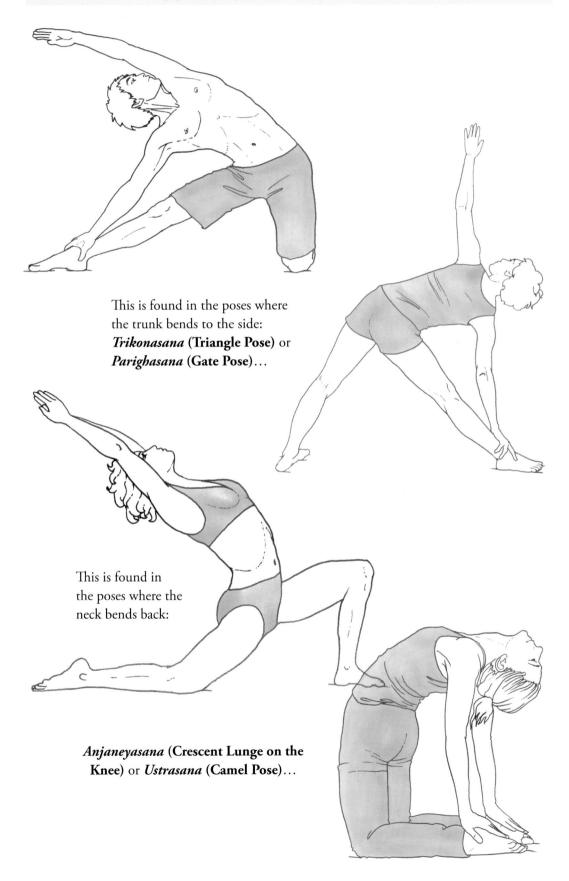

This is found in the poses where
the trunk bends to the side:
Trikonasana (**Triangle Pose**) or
Parighasana (**Gate Pose**)…

This is found in
the poses where the
neck bends back:

Anjaneyasana (**Crescent Lunge on the
Knee**) or *Ustrasana* (**Camel Pose**)…

"Double muscle" contraction

In movements where the trunk curves starting from a vertical position, we have just seen that gravity is the force that produces the movement.

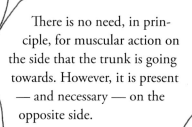

There is no need, in principle, for muscular action on the side that the trunk is going towards. However, it is present — and necessary — on the opposite side.

But we can, nevertheless, choose to contract on the side where we curve. As if it were this contraction that produced the action.

This contraction is then *added to the force of gravity*: in this case it takes twice the contraction as on the opposite side, to hold both the weight of the leaning trunk as well as the contractile action added to this weight.

What is the value of working in this way?

• For one thing, contraction of the concave side will make the action more precise.

• For another, the greater amount of contractions around the moving region builds up a localized "coating."

• The contraction-related blood flow is more significant: there is more micro-circulation.

On the other hand, working in this way has disadvantages:

• the contractions tighten the intervertebral joints more intensely…

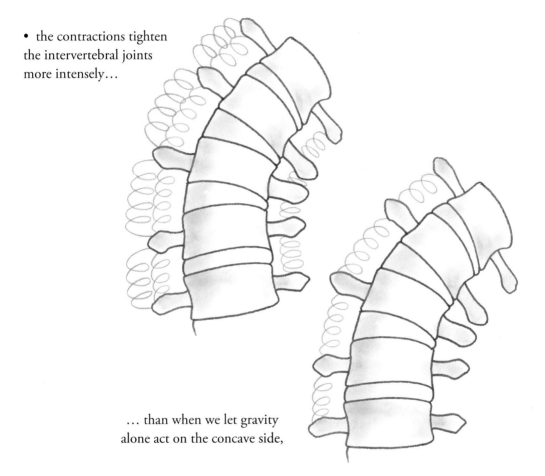

… than when we let gravity alone act on the concave side,

• and — very important — mentioning the muscular action on the concave side should never make us forget that contraction is most indispensable (and most protective) on the convex side, in the opposite direction that we curve.

Contraction may involve muscle in all its states of *length*

A contracting muscle tries to shorten itself. But it is not necessarily in its short position at the beginning of the contraction. Its points of insertion can be very *distant*, or on the contrary, *very close*. Here we take the example of the gluteus maximums (AOM, p. 249) in three different poses.

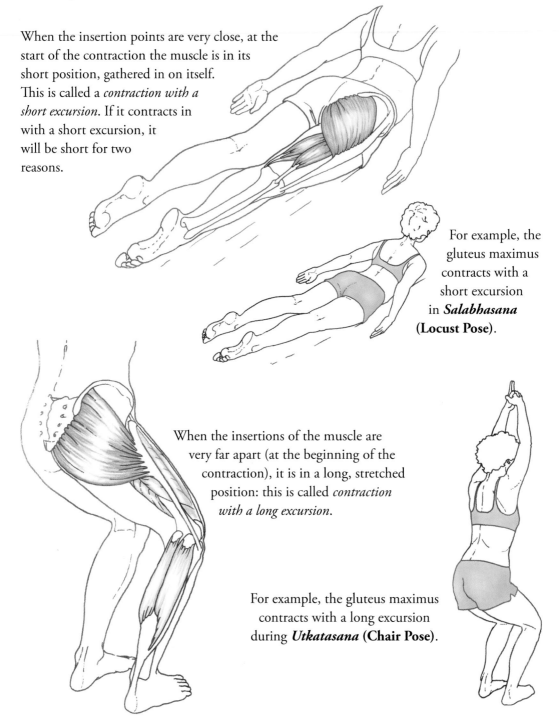

When the insertion points are very close, at the start of the contraction the muscle is in its short position, gathered in on itself. This is called a *contraction with a short excursion*. If it contracts in with a short excursion, it will be short for two reasons.

For example, the gluteus maximus contracts with a short excursion in *Salabhasana* (**Locust Pose**).

When the insertions of the muscle are very far apart (at the beginning of the contraction), it is in a long, stretched position: this is called *contraction with a long excursion*.

For example, the gluteus maximus contracts with a long excursion during *Utkatasana* (**Chair Pose**).

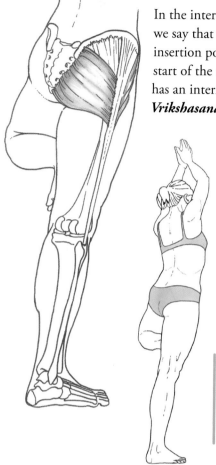

In the intermediate position between these two excursions, we say that the muscle has an intermediate excursion. Its insertion points are neither far apart nor stretched at the start of the contraction. For example, the gluteus maximus has an intermediate excursion for the supporting leg in *Vrikshasana* (**Tree Pose**).

Please note, the types of excursions and the types of contractions can be combined. A muscle can work in concentric, eccentric, or static contraction in all types of excursions.

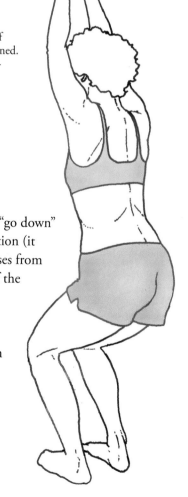

If we take the example of *Utkatasana* (**Chair Pose**): when we "go down" to assume the pose, the gluteus maximus is in *eccentric* contraction (it "puts on the brakes" during the descent), and progressively passes from an intermediate excursion (a little stretched at the beginning of the descent) to a long excursion.

When we come up from the pose, the gluteus maximus is in *concentric* contraction, and it passes from a long excursion to an intermediate excursion.

We can therefore see that the excursion and the types of contraction are continuously combined.

Three types of reflexes present in yoga

A reflex is an unconscious and involuntary action that is done in response to a stimulus.

Many actions in the body are reflexes, that is to say that they are done without being decided on or paid attention to.

Myotatic reflex

Also known as *stretch reflex,* it is triggered when the muscle is stretched by a fast and not very intense lengthening. It causes contraction in the same muscle that is stretched. Thus, the muscle acts against its own stretching.

This reflex, present in all muscles, protects the muscle by preventing it from being stretched by overly-intense situations that could hurt it. It also serves as a base for what is called *muscle tone.* This reflex is based in the spinal cord, even though its circuit is connected to the higher centers of the nervous system.

In yoga, when you want to relax a muscle, particularly in order to stretch it, *you should avoid fast movements.*

Inverse myotatic reflex (Golgi tendon reflex)

This second type of reflex functions in opposition to the first type. It is triggered when the muscle is stretched by a slow and sustained lengthening. It causes relaxation (more or less significant) of the same muscle that is being stretched. The muscle is therefore allowed to extend.

In yoga, this reflex is solicited when your reach the limit of stretching during a pose, and you wait a few seconds: the muscle is then stretched within the limit of its normal length.

From this we should remember that *when you want to relax or stretch a muscle, it is advisable to work with slow movements.*

Reciprocal inhibition reflex

This third type functions with two different muscles that have opposing actions. When one muscle contracts, its antagonist relaxes.

Please note: *this phenomenon does not occur in the non-contractile part of the muscle.*

If a muscle like the hamstring is shortened by a shrinking of its aponeurosis (see p. 16), this reflex is not what will allow it to gain length.

A few words that sometimes cause confusion

These two pages present words that are commonly used in the language of bodywork technique, and in particular yoga. They take on a particular meaning depending on the context, which is not the same from one situation to another. The following lines therefore clarify the meaning given here to these words.

Tense muscle or muscle placed in tension

When you read in this book that a muscle is "tensed," or when it talks about a muscle's "tension," this means that, like a cable, it is placed in tension by the situation which is presented. This tension will not necessarily go far enough to stretch it, but at a minimum, it will place it in its long position.

Please note that the words "tense" and "tension" are often understood in a different sense: it is sometimes said that a person is "tense" if they cannot relax. In this context, the word "tense" could take on the meaning "too contracted" and could refer to the muscle's state of contraction. This is not the meaning that is used here.

Relaxed muscle

When you read in this book that a muscle is "relaxed," or when it talks about "relaxation" of a muscle, this means that its contractile state is less strong. The word therefore refers to the contractile state of the muscle and not to the act of stretching.

Please note that the word "relaxed" can be understood otherwise: it is sometimes said that an elastic band or a bicycle chain is "relaxed," referring to the object's state of length. This is not the meaning that is used in this book, nor in bodywork more generally.

It can therefore be seen that the words "tense" and "relaxed" do not have the same meaning in daily life that they have in bodywork.

Short muscle

When you read in this book that a muscle is "short," this can have several different meanings.

• A muscle can be "short" because *its size is small, anatomically.*

For example, the pectoralis minor is a "short" muscle.

• A muscle can be called "short" or "too short" because it lacks length; *it has shortened.* This is often the case, for example, with the hamstring muscles. Here the word "short" therefore has a very different meaning than in the preceding case, a meaning which is often applicable to muscles of an anatomically long size.

We can also talk of "retracted" muscles, but this has a pathological connotation.

• A muscle can be called "short" because its insertion points are momentarily close together, and it is placed in a short position.

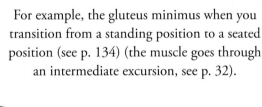

For example, the gluteus minimus when you transition from a standing position to a seated position (see p. 134) (the muscle goes through an intermediate excursion, see p. 32).

Another common source of confusion is that if a muscle is "momentarily short," this does not mean that it is contracted. A muscle can be in a short position — with close insertion points — and be either in complete relaxation or strong contraction.

The meaning of a "short muscle" must therefore be interpreted according to the context.

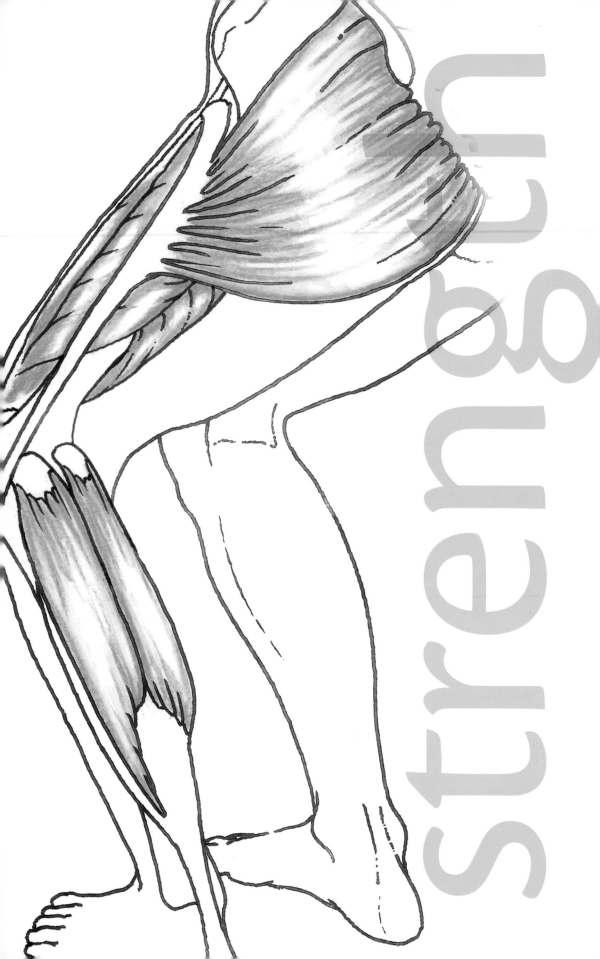

strength

2

Muscle Strength and the Poses

From session to session, yoga strengthens the body.

At one time:

- holding certain poses requires a contraction that is not typical,

- and, in return, this engagement often *strengthens* the muscle or muscles involved.

Muscle strength is not always present in yoga. Some poses require none, and some require only a small amount. In others, *the aspect of muscle strength completely dominates the experience.*

Some poses will require you to develop strength in one precise muscle, without which it cannot be executed, or without which there will be risks. Muscular strength occupies a very different role from one pose to another. The muscle will sometimes protect a joint or a nerve, sometimes it will orient a bone, sometimes it will support a body part, sometimes it will suspend one…

This chapter offers a journey of muscle strength observation and experience through ten yoga poses.

Observations on muscle strength

For a muscle, its available strength varies, depending on *whether it usually exercises its contraction more or less frequently.*

If a muscle does not contract often, it tends to lose volume and strength. It is said to *atrophy.*

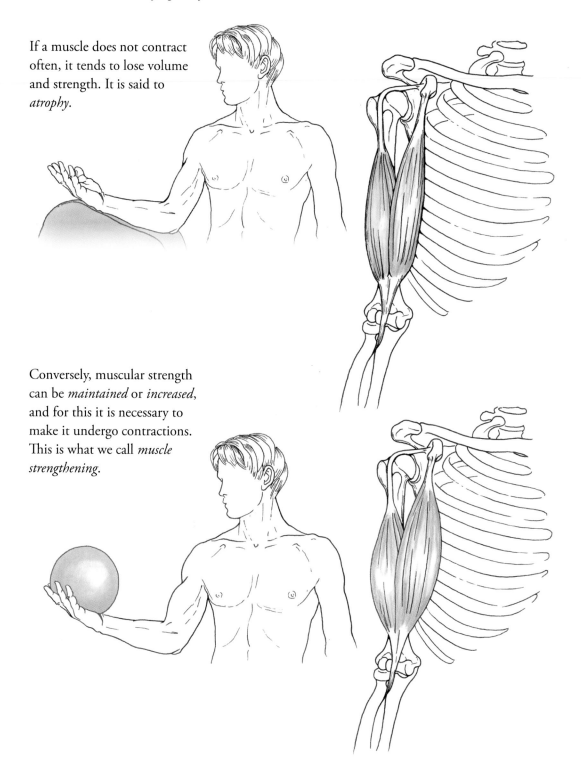

Conversely, muscular strength can be *maintained* or *increased,* and for this it is necessary to make it undergo contractions. This is what we call *muscle strengthening.*

This process is present in yoga, but *not only in yoga*, and *not always in yoga*.

- **Not only in yoga:**

a number of wellness methods offer muscle strengthening programs in the areas of fitness, sports training, methods like Pilates, etc.

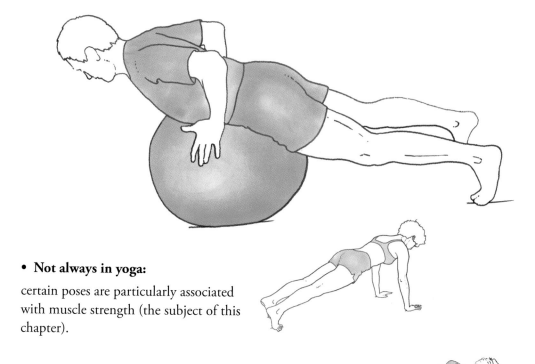

- **Not always in yoga:**

certain poses are particularly associated with muscle strength (the subject of this chapter).

But, in certain other poses, this is not the aim, and we instead seek relaxation (Chapter 3)

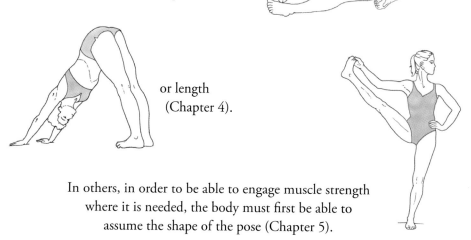

or length
(Chapter 4).

In others, in order to be able to engage muscle strength where it is needed, the body must first be able to assume the shape of the pose (Chapter 5).

It is useful to know how to recognize if a pose requires muscle strength, if it increases this strength (if it can — or cannot— act as a muscle strengthener), if it strengthens a lot or a little, and, better still, which muscles it strengthens.

In order for a muscle to be strengthened, it must *work against a resistance that is greater than usual.*

1) What is *resistance*?

It is *all the force that opposes that of the muscle*, and which can be very diverse.

This may be:

• the weight of body parts (for example, the weight of the arm opposes the contraction of the deltoid muscle).

The heavier or more numerous the parts of the body to be mobilized or maintained are, the stronger the resistance, and the more intense the muscular action must be.

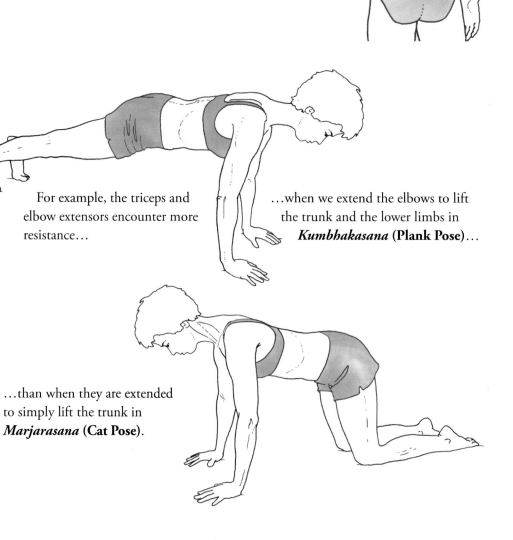

For example, the triceps and elbow extensors encounter more resistance…

…when we extend the elbows to lift the trunk and the lower limbs in *Kumbhakasana* (**Plank Pose**)…

…than when they are extended to simply lift the trunk in *Marjarasana* (**Cat Pose**).

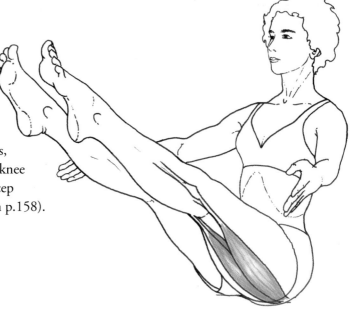

• the tensioning of antagonist muscles. For example, when we want to raise the thighs in *Navasana* **(Boat Pose)** with straight knees, the muscle tension behind the knee resists the action of the quadricep muscle (see detailed analysis on p.158).

• the lifting of supplemental weights, which is not often found in yoga.

• an action brought about by another person or by a device, which is sometimes encountered in yoga (as in Acroyoga).

• the action of an antagonist muscle. This is found in settings with a joint action of two muscles that unite opposing forces to stabilize a bone or region.

For example, in *Kumbhakasana* **(Plank Pose)**, the serratus anterior muscle, abductor of the scapulae, contracts at the same time as the rhomboid, adductor of these same scapulae, in order to stabilize them on the thorax.

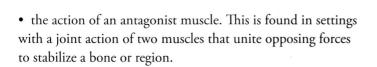

2) Resistance that is *greater than the usual*

For someone who does not practice much physical activity (who walks on flat ground, sits, and stands), the simple act of climbing a staircase imposes resistance on the muscles of the lower limbs that is greater than any of their usual actions.

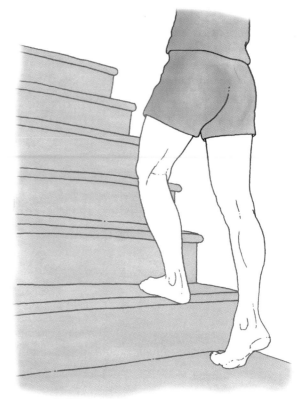

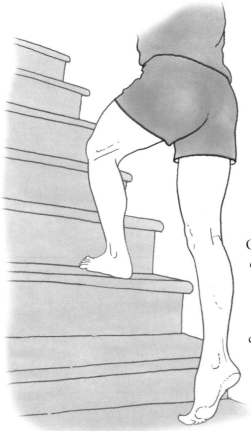

On the other hand, for a person accustomed to climbing several staircases each day, the act of climbing one does not present greater resistance than usual: it would be necessary to increase the number of steps, or climb them two by two, or carry loads, or climb more quickly…

It can thus be seen that the resistance which must be offered for muscle strengthening is quite variable from one person to another. It will not be the same in a retirement home as it is in a professional sports training club, and this is true for any yoga session.

Sometimes, a pose cannot be taken because the muscular strength necessary to realize or hold it is insufficient.

For example, lifting the trunk by pushing through the limbs in *Chakrasana* (**Bridge Pose**) requires a lot of strength in the root muscles (muscles of the shoulder girdle, but also the deltoids for the arms, and the pelvic muscles for the legs). It also takes a lot of strength in the middle of the limbs (the triceps brachii to extend the elbows, and the quadriceps to extend the knees).

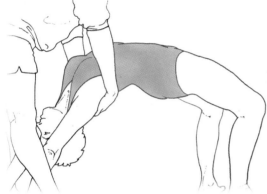

If this strength is lacking, the trunk stays on the ground. The form of the pose could be taken with an aide lifting the thorax, but not through the muscular strength of the person herself (see an analysis of this pose on p. 166).

It is therefore necessary to prepare the pose by strengthening all the muscles that have just been mentioned (but also — and this is another subject — by "lifting" all the anatomical obstacles that prevent it from being assumed comfortably).

Should we strengthen them with the pose itself? Or through other poses that target this or that muscle in the series? It is possible. But it is not always necessary: we can strengthen the muscles of the lower limbs by climbing (or descending) the stairs. We can strengthen those of the upper limbs by carrying loads.

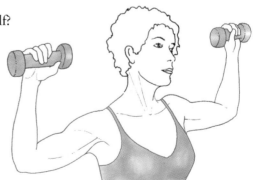

From this example we can see that the strength necessary for certain poses can be prepared for by strengthening during yoga but also outside the realm of yoga poses. In this book, both cases will be presented.

The following pages will present ten poses:

- The first seven primarily require muscle strength, and their main effect is to develop this strength, without necessitating any particular flexibility.

- The last three require targeted strength in certain muscles.

10 Themed Explanation Sheets: Poses Discussed

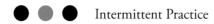

Intermittent Practice

Strengthen the muscles in the back of the body in
Utkatasana (Chair Pose)

With the *feet flat* and the *back inclined*

This pose requires you to send your body in two different directions: the lower limbs descend in triple flexion (the hips, knees, and ankles), and the trunk and arms rise up and forward as much as possible. Practicing the pose develops strength in the posterior muscles as well as in the quadriceps, both essential for keeping the body vertical. We can detail each relevant area with some exercises that work them partially.

Crouch slowly: starting from a standing position with feet parallel, go down in slow motion while bending the knees.

Feel how the gluteus maximus (AOM, p. 249) contracts in order to hold the pelvis, the quadriceps and triceps (AOM, pp. 238 and 292) and to support the knees and ankles.

As you descend, these three "giant" muscles will work more and more, and in a position that is increasingly stretched.

Slowly lower the trunk: start again from a standing position with the feet parallel, now lean the trunk forward in slow motion without bending it, starting at the hips.

If you place your fingers in the middle of your back, you will feel the back muscles (AOM, p. 78) contract more and more — and increasingly widely — as you go down. The contraction spreads upwards to the whole back of your neck.

Feel the abdominals: lower the trunk again while placing the hands against your stomach. Feel the strength in your abdominals (AOM, pp. 94-97) intensify as you descend. This contraction essentially serves to contain the internal organs, and not to hold the position.

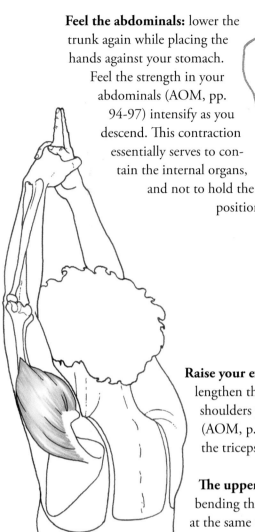

Raise your extended arms: still in the same position, now lengthen the arms, elbows extended. In the back of your shoulders you now feel the posterior deltoid muscles (AOM, p. 132), and in the back of the arms you can feel the triceps muscles extending the elbows.

The upper and lower body together: now practice bending the knees, tilting the trunk, and raising the arms at the same time. All the muscular actions discussed above coexist in your body. This is a powerful cladding.

We find this in part in other poses: *Salabhasana* (**Locust Pose**), *Surya Namaskara* (**Sun Salutation**) and *Virabhadrasna* (**Warrior Pose**)

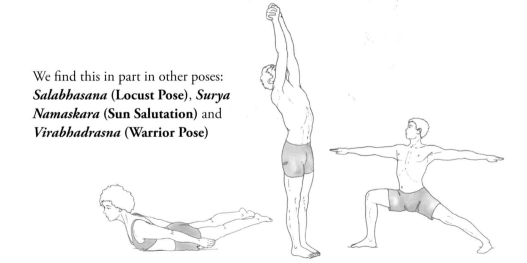

Strengthen the muscles of the lower limbs in
Utkatasana (Chair Pose)

On the balls of your feet.

This pose involves balancing while simultaneously bending the knees and ankles. It requires strength in the main joints of the lower limbs. Practicing it will provide you with stable ankles and knees in many other poses. The details can be discovered through some preparatory exercises.

Rise onto the balls of your feet: place yourself in a standing position, near a stable object that you can hold onto.

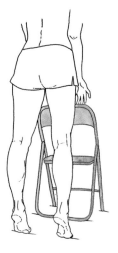

Rise onto the balls of your feet. This engages your triceps surae (AOM, p. 292).

Feel how the ankle tends to tilt laterally, especially outward. This tendency is much stronger on the balls of the feet because the bones are less nested and the ligaments relaxed. You must therefore hold the foot in place with muscular actions.

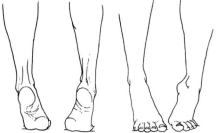

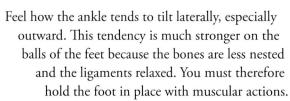

Stabilize the ankles: first allow the foot to move laterally. This changes the support of the foot, which is now found on the outer part of your forefoot while the big toe and fleshy area behind it barely rest on the ground. Now try to bring the support back to this latter area. To do so, feel the action on the outside of the leg, along the fibula. These are the peroneus muscles (AOM, p. 288), which complement the powerful action of the triceps surae in the calf, as well as that of many small muscles in the foot itself.

Bend and stabilize the knee: while standing, bend the knees a little. This position relaxes the knee ligaments, which are less stable than when they are stretched. Then move to one knee. Stay balanced, moving your arms or the other leg: this requires the action of all your knee muscles, particularly the quadriceps (AOM, p. 238) and the hamstring muscles (AOM, p. 242).

Knees and ankles together: now practice bending your knees and rising onto the balls of your feet at the same time. For the four joints, you need a muscular action. But in addition, you have to balance the hips, and for this you engage the gluteus muscles (medius and maximus).

Utkatasana also strengthens, but with less intensity, the anterior deltoid muscles (for lifting the arms), the tricep muscles (for extending the elbows), the extensor muscles of the wrists and fingers, and for holding the trunk, the dorsal and abdominal muscles.

We find this partly in other poses: *Anjaneyasana* (**Crescent Lunge on the Knee**), *Virabhadrasna* (**Warrior Pose**), and the **standing balancing poses**, particularly those on one foot.

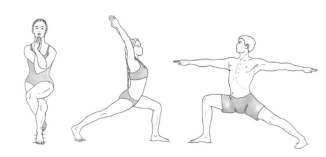

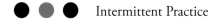 Intermittent Practice

Strengthen the muscles of the upper limbs in *Bakasana* (Crow Pose)

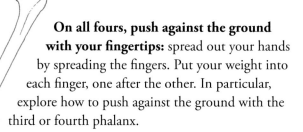

This pose involves bringing the body to the forearms and hands. It is mainly balanced on the supporting arms, whose muscles must stabilize the major joints.

We can discover them through some preliminary exercises.

On all fours, push against the ground with your fingertips: spread out your hands by spreading the fingers. Put your weight into each finger, one after the other. In particular, explore how to push against the ground with the third or fourth phalanx.

In doing so, you strengthen the flexor muscles of the fingers (AOM, p. 176). The deep flexor goes to the third phalanx, the superficial flexor to the second.

Note: the two drawings show a simplified model of these muscles and not the detailed anatomy of the tendons.

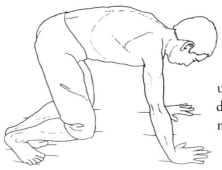

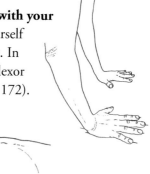

Push against the ground with your full hand: now support yourself using the palms of your hands. In doing so, you strengthen the flexor muscle of the wrist (AOM, p. 172).

Push from the elbows: Bend your elbows a little. Try to extend them — but without realizing the action — to create and build your support. You thus contract the powerful muscles located at the backs of the arms: the triceps (AOM, p. 148).

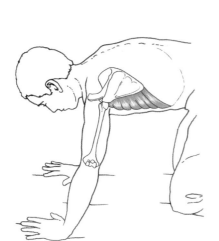

Push from the shoulder: now try to spread your scapulae. This makes them slide towards the front of the thorax — or, since you are on all fours, towards the ground.

Act as if the pressure in your hands came directly from your scapulae. You are strengthening a powerful muscle situated on the side of the thorax: the serratus anterior muscle (AOM, p. 120).

Now take the pose by bringing your bent knees as high as possible on the backs of your arms. Bring your weight onto your hands, repelling the ground by combining all the actions discussed above.

Then, lift your feet up one at a time.

We find this in part in other poses:
Bhujangasana **(Cobra Pose),**
Kumbhakasana **(Plank Pose),**
Purvottanasana **(Upward Plank Pose).**

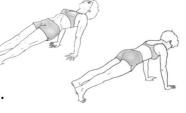

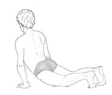

Strengthen the anterior musculature in
Kumbhakasana (Plank Pose)

This pose orients the body towards the ground. To
properly align it requires strength in the front
of the trunk. Here too, we can practice it
partially.

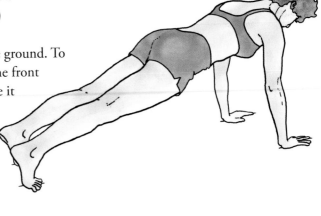

Support the space between the ribs and the pelvis: go onto all
fours. Come a little forward so as to support yourself more on the
hands than the knees. Then, conversely, come back a little so as to
support yourself more on the knees than the hands.

Repeat this weight transfer several times.
Throughout the movement, feel how between
your sternum and pelvis your trunk remains
stable. To that end, contract the abdominals
(AOM, p. 97) and the dorsal muscles, which
synergistically hold the ribcage-pelvis distance,
and support the internal organs
like a hammock.

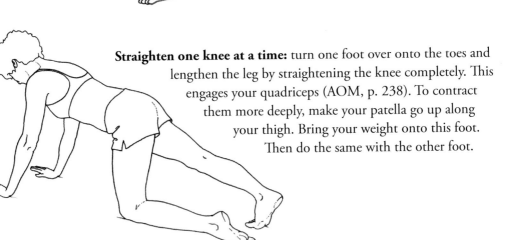

Straighten one knee at a time: turn one foot over onto the toes and
lengthen the leg by straightening the knee completely. This
engages your quadriceps (AOM, p. 238). To contract
them more deeply, make your patella go up along
your thigh. Bring your weight onto this foot.
Then do the same with the other foot.

Straighten both knees: turn both feet over onto the toes, knees straight.

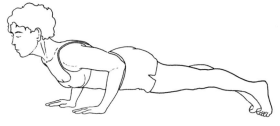

Now feel the serratus anterior muscles engage on the sides of the thorax (AOM, p. 120).

Keep the scapula well glued to the body and in front of the shoulder in order to direct the arm towards the ground (the pectoralis major, AOM, p. 130, and the anterior deltoid, AOM, p. 132).

All these muscles work vigorously to prevent the trunk from lowering to the ground. Added to this is the contraction of the triceps, at the back of the arms, to extend the elbows.

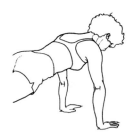

If your elbows can hyperextend, avoid placing yourself in hyperextension because then there will be no more action of the triceps.

Balance the pelvis: your pelvis tends to fall towards the ground. To prevent this, you must contract your hip flexors (AOM, p. 252). But if these muscles act too strongly, they will bring your pelvis up so that you are no longer in rectilinear head-feet alignment.

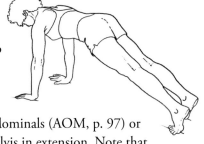

Place the pelvis in extension: contract either your abdominals (AOM, p. 97) or your gluteus maximus (AOM, p. 249) to place your pelvis in extension. Note that this action goes in the opposite direction of the previous one. You now forcefully contract the muscles in front of and behind your pelvis.

Hold the internal organs: you still have to keep the internal organs from falling by using the abdominals, which act like a hammock.

We find this in part in other poses: *Vasisthasana* **(Side Plank Pose)**, *Ardha Pincha Mayurasana* **(Dolphin Pose)**, and *Marjaryasana* **(Cat Pose)**.

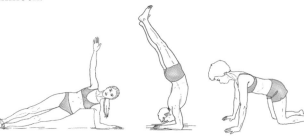

● ◐ ●   Intermittent Practice

Strengthen the anterior and posterior musculature in
Navasana (Boat Pose)

or in *Supta Konasana* (Reclining Angle Pose)

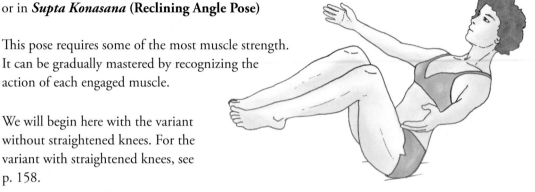

This pose requires some of the most muscle strength. It can be gradually mastered by recognizing the action of each engaged muscle.

We will begin here with the variant without straightened knees. For the variant with straightened knees, see p. 158.

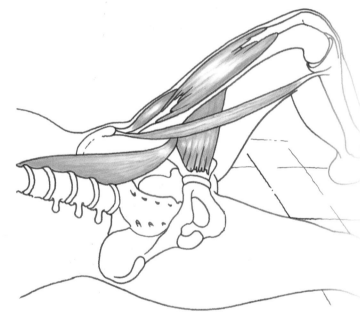

Flex the thighs: lie on your back or rest on your elbows. Bring one thigh into flexion, letting the knee bend.

Identify the action of the hip flexors: the psoas, whose action can be felt deep in the bottom of the trunk, and the iliacus, whose action is felt from inside the pelvis (AOM, p. 234).

Also the tensor fasciae latae (AOM, p. 248), the gluteus minimus (AOM, p. 236), the sartorius muscle (AOM, p. 241), whose contractions can be felt under the anterior superior iliac spine.

Identify flexion of the pelvis and stabilize the pelvis: lift the thighs simultaneously. Feel how the actions of the muscles noted above cause the pelvis to tilt further towards the coccyx, as it flexes.

Stabilize the pelvis: to keep the pelvis in place, engage the rectus abdominis muscle of the abdomen.

Lean the trunk back: place yourself now in a seated position, on the tops of your ischia, your knees bent and feet resting on the ground. Keeping the trunk straight, go back a little as a single head-neck-trunk block. Immediately feel a strong action in your rectus abdominis muscles, which holds your trunk (your ribs are secured to your pelvis).

Straighten the pelvis: also feel how this strong abdominal action tends to roll your pelvis back behind your ischia.

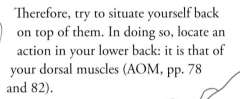

Therefore, try to situate yourself back on top of them. In doing so, locate an action in your lower back: it is that of your dorsal muscles (AOM, pp. 78 and 82).

Now take the full *Navasana* (**Boat Pose)** and feel the cumulative and powerful action of all the muscles detailed on this page. To these are added the anterior deltoid muscles (for raising the arms) and the triceps muscles (for extending the elbows).

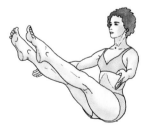

For an even more intense pose, see p. 158 for the version with straight knees.

We find this in part in other poses: *Purvottanasana* (**Upward Plank Pose).**

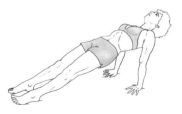

● ● ●   Intermittent Practice

Simultaneously strengthen the anterior and posterior muscles in
Purvottanasana (Upward Plank Pose)

This pose places the body in balance between the hands and the feet, facing upward.

It powerfully strengthens the posterior muscles, and in particular the backward movement of the shoulders. Here we find several of the muscles seen in previous poses.

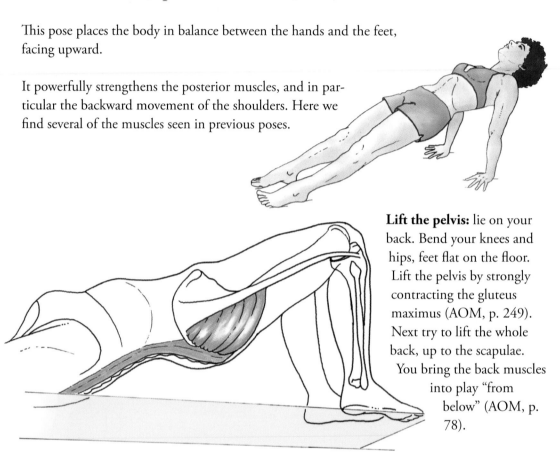

Lift the pelvis: lie on your back. Bend your knees and hips, feet flat on the floor. Lift the pelvis by strongly contracting the gluteus maximus (AOM, p. 249). Next try to lift the whole back, up to the scapulae. You bring the back muscles into play "from below" (AOM, p. 78).

Support yourself on your arms: Sit down and place your hands a little behind your pelvis. Support yourself on your hands and let them carry the weight of your trunk. Try to push against the ground (find all the steps for this support on p. 52).

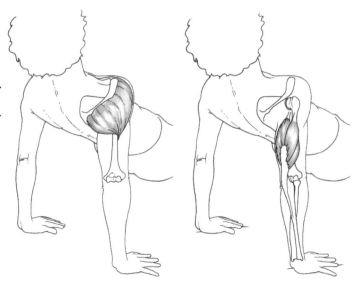

Bring the shoulders back: try to bring the scapulae together, as they tend to move apart. For this, you contract the rhomboid muscles (AOM, p. 123).

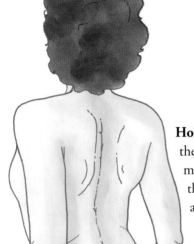

Hollow your back: extend the shoulder-squeezing movement by engaging the dorsal muscles "from above."

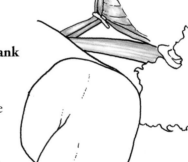

Next take the full *Purvottanasana* **(Upward Plank Pose),** aiming for rectilinear alignment starting from the feet. For this you add a contraction of the abdominal muscles that maintain the distance between the ribcage and the pelvis. You also contract the muscles that prevent the head and neck from going back: the sternocleidomastoid muscle (AOM, p. 88) and the suprahyoid and infrahyoid muscles (AOM, p. 87).*

*The suprahyoid and infrahyoid muscles, groups of several small muscles found at the front of the neck, are described in detail in my book *Anatomy of Voice,* pp. 180-184.

We find this in part in other poses:
Ustrasana **(Camel Pose)** and
Navasana **(Boat Pose).**

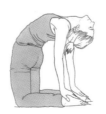

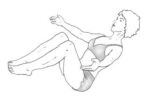

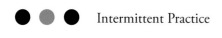 Intermittent Practice

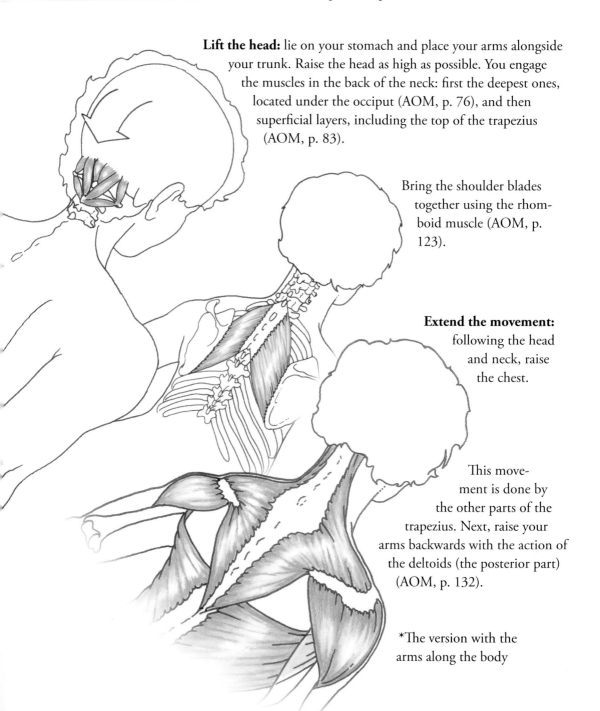

Strengthen the posterior muscles
in *Salabhasana** (Locust Pose)

This pose straightens the entire head-neck-trunk axis, as well as the legs. It powerfully strengthens the posterior muscles, including the gluteus muscles. Here we find several of the muscles seen in previous poses.

Lift the head: lie on your stomach and place your arms alongside your trunk. Raise the head as high as possible. You engage the muscles in the back of the neck: first the deepest ones, located under the occiput (AOM, p. 76), and then superficial layers, including the top of the trapezius (AOM, p. 83).

Bring the shoulder blades together using the rhomboid muscle (AOM, p. 123).

Extend the movement: following the head and neck, raise the chest.

This movement is done by the other parts of the trapezius. Next, raise your arms backwards with the action of the deltoids (the posterior part) (AOM, p. 132).

*The version with the arms along the body

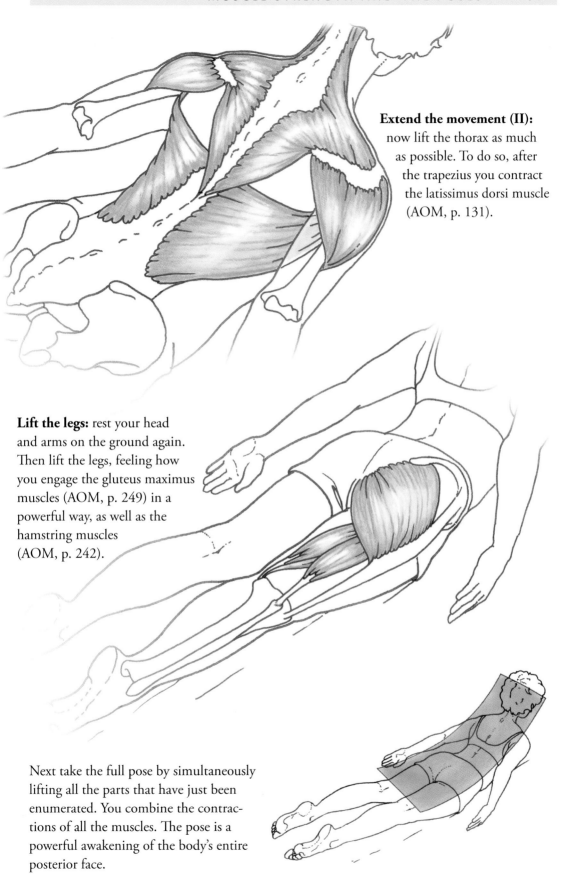

Extend the movement (II): now lift the thorax as much as possible. To do so, after the trapezius you contract the latissimus dorsi muscle (AOM, p. 131).

Lift the legs: rest your head and arms on the ground again. Then lift the legs, feeling how you engage the gluteus maximus muscles (AOM, p. 249) in a powerful way, as well as the hamstring muscles (AOM, p. 242).

Next take the full pose by simultaneously lifting all the parts that have just been enumerated. You combine the contractions of all the muscles. The pose is a powerful awakening of the body's entire posterior face.

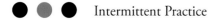 Intermittent Practice

Strengthen muscles that are often weak in
Matsyasana (Fish Pose)

This pose strongly extends the anterior and upper parts of the body. For this to be achieved harmoniously, you must almost completely suspend the head, which bears almost no weight on the ground: the front of the neck is thus in a position that lengthens all the anterior structures (ligaments, muscles, but also internal organs and glands). This opening spreads to the regions of the shoulders and thorax.

So as to (almost) not rest on the head, you must *transfer the support of the upper body to the forearms.* This requires muscular strength in several areas: for *extending the elbows,* for *keeping the arms back behind the trunk,* for *keeping the scapulae close together* and for *keeping the trunk straight.*

The muscles that do this have in common the fact that they are located on the posterior part of the body. However, in the upper body, strength is not equal between the muscles that close the arms/cross them forward, and those which, on the contrary, open the arms/bring them backward: the latter muscles are, overall, half as strong. In **Matsyasana**, it is these muscles that are engaged intensely. This is very useful for strengthening an area that opens the thorax. We can observe these muscles one after the other.

The scapulae are squeezed together behind the thorax, as a result of the trapezius and the rhomboids: in setting up the pose, you bring together the shoulder blades, which engages the rhomboid deeply (AOM, p. 123), and the trapezius, more superficially (AOM, p. 124). If these muscles are too weak, the arms do not stay "close" to the body, and it is difficult to support the trunk.

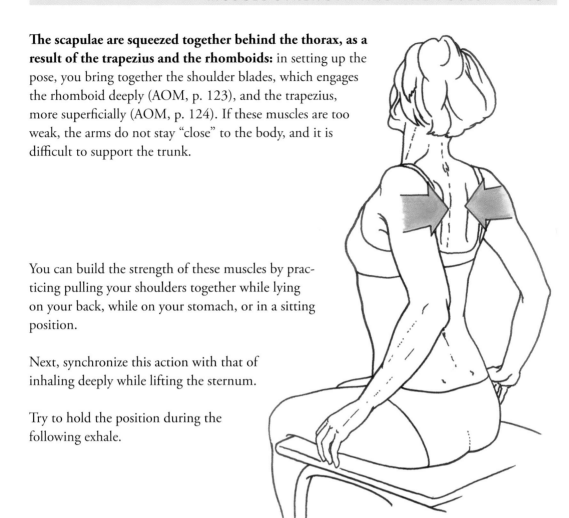

You can build the strength of these muscles by practicing pulling your shoulders together while lying on your back, while on your stomach, or in a sitting position.

Next, synchronize this action with that of inhaling deeply while lifting the sternum.

Try to hold the position during the following exhale.

The thorax hollows in back, as a result of the dorsal muscles (AOM, p. 78), which straighten the spine. If they are too weak, the thorax will not turn over enough to allow the neck and head to be suspended from it. You can build their strength, for example, with *Salabhasana* **(Locust Pose)**, see p. 60. Here too, synchronize this action with that of inhaling deeply while lifting the sternum.

○ ○ ○ *Continued…*

Extension of the elbows as a result of the triceps (AOM, p. 148): we try to push the forearms and hands against the ground, to straighten the arm from the pressure on the forearm. The action is that of the triceps brachii (AOM, p. 148). If it is not strong enough, the arm will not be well-anchored to the ground.

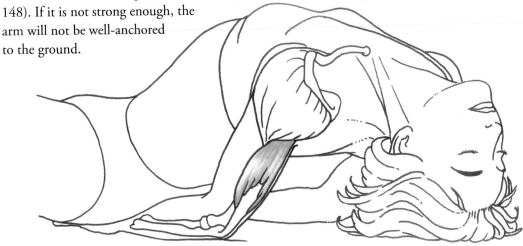

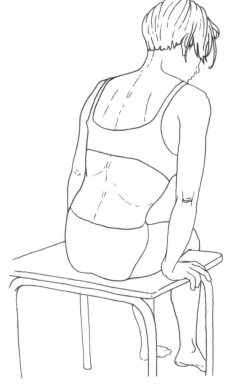

You can build the strength of your triceps, in advance, with any situation involving support with the hands — elbows a little bent — such as *Kumbhakasana* (**Plank Pose**).

(**Warning:** the elbows must not be straightened, since there is then a bone wedge in the elbow and thus no more contraction of the triceps.)

The arms behind the trunk, as a result of the posterior deltoids: the deltoid muscle (AOM, p. 132) can have very different actions.

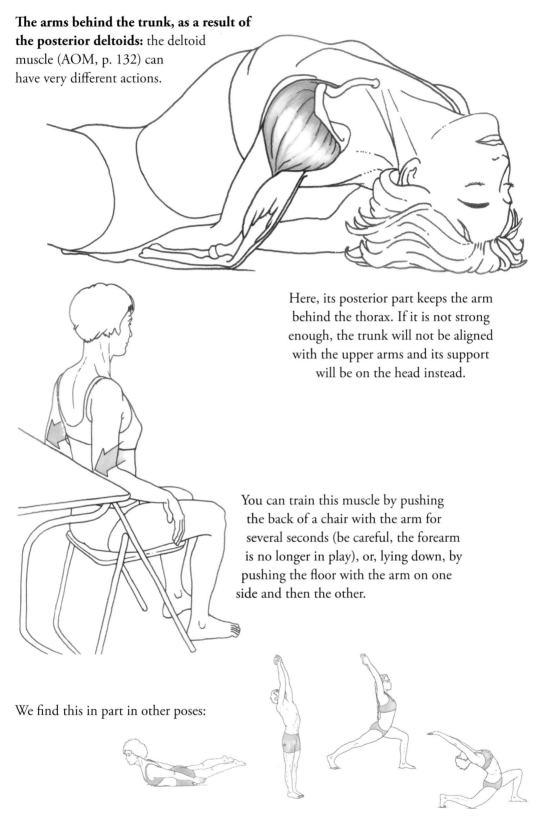

Here, its posterior part keeps the arm behind the thorax. If it is not strong enough, the trunk will not be aligned with the upper arms and its support will be on the head instead.

You can train this muscle by pushing the back of a chair with the arm for several seconds (be careful, the forearm is no longer in play), or, lying down, by pushing the floor with the arm on one side and then the other.

We find this in part in other poses:

Salabhasana **(Locust Pose),** *Anjaneyasana* **(Crescent Lunge on the Knee),** and *Ashta Chandrasana* **(Crescent Moon Pose).**

● ● ● Practice at the End

Strengthen the longus colli in
Sirsasana (Headstand)

This pose requires you to balance the weight of almost the entire body on the cervical vertebrae, whose vertebral bodies are three times smaller than those of the lumbar vertebrae.

This action requires precision.

Before lifting the trunk and legs, you must first balance the cervical vertebrae one on top of the other. For one thing, *they must not tilt laterally*: the contractions of the scalenes, on each side of the neck (AOM, p. 86), ensure this equilibrium.

For another, *the weight must be received by the vertebral bodies and the discs,* and not by the small posterior joints of the vertebrae. Therefore, the structure of the cervical vertebrae must not go into hyperextension (arching) or into flexion: it must be *completely stabilized in front and in back.*

The hands placed behind the occiput keep the head and neck from rolling into flexion. Continue keeping the cervical vertebrae from going too far into extension through an action in the direction of flexion, which must remain measured and distributed along the vertebrae.

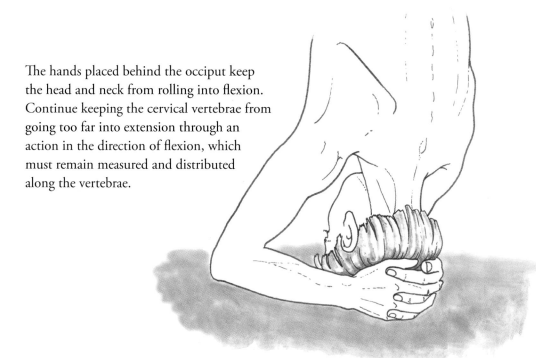

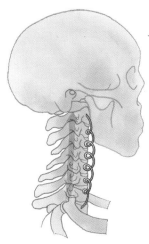

A pair of deep muscles come in just in front of the cervical vertebrae: the longus colli (AOM, p. 84). Their contraction occurs very close to the vertebrae, straightening the cervical curvature and straightening the alignment. Because of their numerous bundles, their contraction occurs with precision: the cervical vertebrae do not "hollow," and the neck forms a powerful pillar, responsive to the burden from the head to its base, as if the head was actively repelling the ground.

Find the contraction of the longus colli: certain exercises allow us to find this muscle, in preparation for the headstand*:

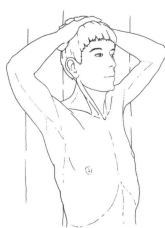

1) Lie on your back with your hips, knees, and ankles bent and your feet flat on the floor. Bring your hands, fingers crossed, to the very top of your head (neither to the front, which will make you flex the neck, nor to the back, which will make you lift your chin).

Gradually bend your elbows, and push your hands on your skull. This pressure is similar to that of the ground, that is to say that for the moment it is horizontal. In return, search for a pushing of the head that responds to that of the hands, and which comes from an action in the cervical vertebrae. *Note:* do not do this by making a double-chin (that is a different muscular strategy), but let it come from your neck instead.

First work with very light pressure (a few hundred grams), before increasing the intensity a little at a time (up to several kilos).

At first, practice on the ground to align the spine.

2) Later, you will repeat the same movement while *standing*, beginning by placing your back against a wall and maintaining contact with this wall (it isn't for pushing against, but should be used as an alignment guide).

3) Later still, when you feel that your neck has acquired the necessary strength to direct this pushing, you can move away from the wall. Finally, you will discover these sensations while setting up *Sirasana* **(Headstand).**

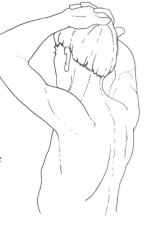

*These strengthening exercises should be preceded by an alignment or re-alignment of the neck. If you feel that you need a support, place it under the nape of your neck, and avoid practicing the headstand as long as the support is needed. (See p. 206 on the scalene muscles.)

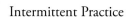

Intermittent Practice

Strengthen the gluteus medius in
Vrikshasana (Tree Pose)

Perched on a single supporting leg, this pose requires adjustment to the position of the pelvis, among others.

When you bring the flat of the foot against the opposite thigh, it feels like you are pressing on it heavily. This support is caused indirectly by the position of the hip (flexion/abduction/external rotation), added to the strong flexion of the knee: this transforms the weight of the whole lower limb (thigh, leg, foot) into horizontal pressure of the foot on the supporting thigh, which tends to become more oblique. At the same time, the pelvis tends to move in three different ways:

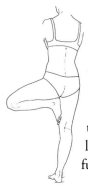

1) The line between the two anterior superior iliac spines is no longer horizontal. It tends to rise on the side of the bent knee, the pelvis pulled along with the thigh that is raised by the hip ligaments. This will not be further explained here.

2) The pelvis is shifted to the outside of the supporting leg. In other words, the angle between the pelvis and the femur is more open towards the outside.

Here a muscle comes in to stabilize it. The gluteus medius (AOM, p. 237) is located at the exterior of the pelvis, on its lateral face. It is a strong abductor of the hip: if the pelvis is fixed, it raises the thigh laterally.

But the action that matters here is the one that occurs when the femur is fixed: it then tilts the pelvis laterally. It can therefore balance it by preventing it from shifting to the outside of the femur.

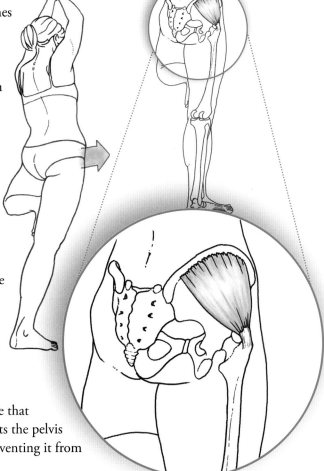

Discover the action of the gluteus medius: in response to the pushing of the foot on the thigh, try to "respond" in the opposite direction, making sure that *your supporting thigh actively repels the foot placed on it.* To bring this about, the alignment must be adjusted.

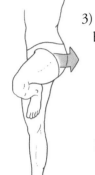

3) The pelvis tends to go back and into flexion,

simultaneously pulled by the bent leg and by the extension of the supporting leg.

A muscular ensemble intervenes here: the gluteus maximus and the pelvic deltoid muscle.

The gluteus maximus (AOM, p. 249) is more superficial than the gluteus medius. It attaches to the back of hip bone and the sacrum, then descends to end at the fascia lata. In front, another muscle (the tensor fasciae latae) also ends on this long fascia.

The three structures together form a group called the *pelvic deltoid muscle* (AOM, p. 250), which, like the gluteus medius, abducts the thigh. But it adds another action: it stabilizes the pelvis by preventing it from moving backwards. The pelvis is brought more in line with the supporting foot.

Prepare for *Vrikshasana* by locating the action of the gluteus maximus: Stand with your feet parallel. Rock the entire body so that it is over the front of the feet (see p. 174) and comes back again. Repeat several times so as to feel the weight-bearing of the back or front of the feet, through a movement that is only in the ankles.

Then, find the same transfer on the front of the feet, by only moving the pelvis (the trunk and head remain vertical to the pelvis). To do so, you must engage the gluteus maximus.

Next, do the same movement but on one leg. When you have mastered this placement of the pelvis, you can combine it with the lateral placement seen above.

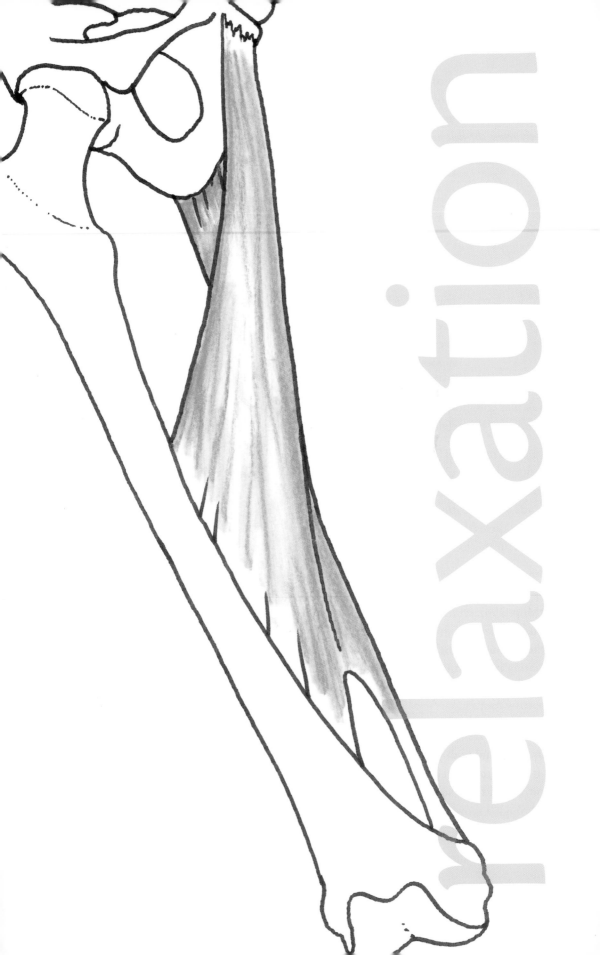

3

Muscle Relaxation in the Poses

As we saw in the preceding chapter, yoga poses sometimes require a lot of strength, both general and targeted.

In a different way, certain poses require knowledge of how to *relax* particular muscles.

One of the benefits of yoga is that it *explores varying states of muscle tone*. Sometimes, "relaxing" certain areas is crucial for holding a pose harmoniously over an extended period of time.

This chapter explores the muscles that should be relaxed in poses that must be held for a long time, such as seated poses and **Shavasana (Corpse Pose)**.

Just as muscular contraction often occurs where we least expect it, muscular relaxation is not always where you expect it to be.

We will also observe how contracting a muscle in the right place facilitates muscular relaxation in the right place.

Observations on muscular relaxation

In order for a muscle to relax, the joint that it
mobilizes can be neither *at risk of dislocation*, nor
in need of support.

1) If there is a risk of dislocation

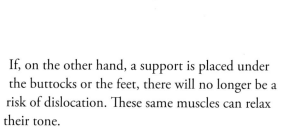

If, for example, a person is suspended by their hands from a trapeze,
the ligaments of the vertebral column are at risk of being distended by
the weight of the trunk.

In these conditions, the muscles of the trunk (dorsal and spinal) cannot
relax: they remain in action in order to *guarantee articular cohesion*.

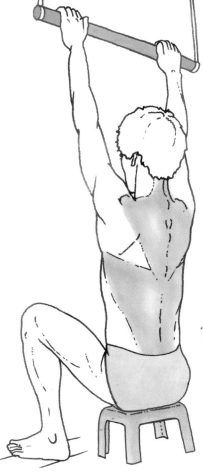

If, on the other hand, a support is placed under
the buttocks or the feet, there will no longer be a
risk of dislocation. These same muscles can relax
their tone.

The muscles are thus ready to react when a situation
threatens to stretch a ligament or, even more simply,
when a ligament is kept in a position of tension —
even moderate — for some time. To more or less
release the muscles, it is necessary to facilitate the
opposite situation.

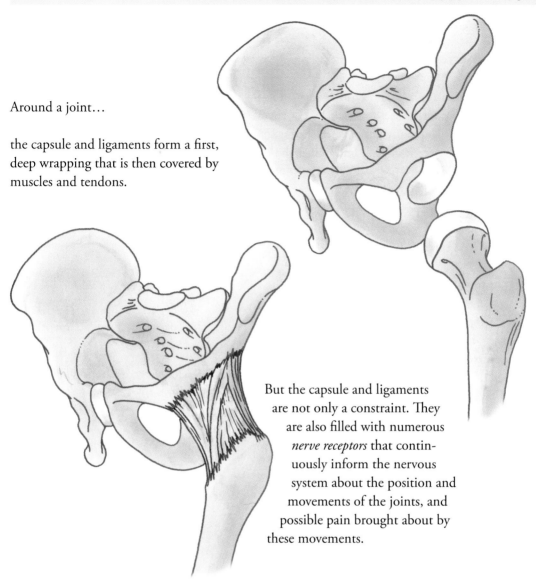

Around a joint…

the capsule and ligaments form a first, deep wrapping that is then covered by muscles and tendons.

But the capsule and ligaments are not only a constraint. They are also filled with numerous *nerve receptors* that continuously inform the nervous system about the position and movements of the joints, and possible pain brought about by these movements.

They are in some ways "warning device" tissues that signal the state of affairs, initiating a contraction on the part of the muscles if the joint is at risk, or even if they are in tension around the joint. This arrangement is beneficial, since it allows the muscles to intervene at the slightest risk of joint dislocation.

The consequence is that, if you want to deeply stretch the muscles of a joint, the ligamental apparatus must be taken out of "warning device" mode, and placed in a state called "ligamentous silence."

Muscular contraction can then decrease.

Articular rest position

For each joint, there is a position where all its ligaments are in an intermediate position and none are very tense. It is called "the articular rest position." Theoretically, in this position the ligament will not warn the nervous system of a need for muscular action. It is in this position that we immobilize the joint when we want to prevent or calm possible inflammation. It is important to understand in order to relax the muscles of the joint. The first explanation sheet of this chapter presents several situations involving the articular rest position.

2) If there is a need for support

If, for example, you are writing at the computer without supporting the elbows, the entire upper-limb, up to the shoulder — which needs support — will be supported by muscle contractions.

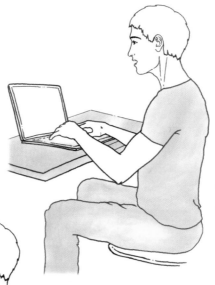

Those of the shoulder (deltoid, supraspinatus) cannot, therefore, relax.

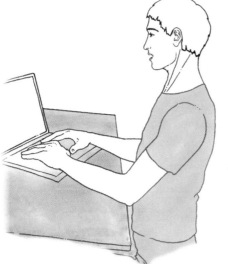

If, however, the elbow and forearm are supported, these muscles can relax their tone.

The situation here is a little different from the previous one: it is not the presence of "risk" that elicits muscular contraction, but rather the necessity of support.

Some schools of yoga, such as Restorative Yoga or certain camps within Iyengar Yoga, focus on placing all or part of the body in a state of relaxation.

It should be noted that this requires setting up facilities and equipment

- that support parts of the body during the poses (such as bolsters, pillows, stools, wedges, blocks, folded mats, etc.). This equipment responds to the "support needs" of the joints, which are no longer necessary to secure through muscular contraction;

- that retain the range of motion in the joints (such as straps, restraints, and blocks, etc.). This equipment responds to the "risk of dislocation," which is anticipated by keeping the joints in non-extreme positions.

It is therefore possible to place the body "in the form of the pose," to give it the benefits of the form (inversion, localized opening), without the assistance of muscular contractions that, usually, are necessary to maintain it.

The effects of this are different: it lacks the muscle strengthening of a pose practiced in an active manner, but it also lacks the joint compression brought about by muscular action.

THE FOLLOWING PAGES will present five poses related to the theme of muscular relaxation. Different questions will arise:

- Does the pose really permit muscular decontraction where it is sought?

- Does the pose require muscular relaxation in a particular part of the body in order for it to be performed correctly?

- Is a modification of the pose necessary in order to allow this relaxation?

- Is this muscular relaxation beneficial for the body?

5 Themed Explanation Sheets: Poses Discussed

Intermittent Practice

Shavasana (Corpse Pose):
Is muscular relaxation totally present?

In this pose, the body is stretched out on its
back, with the limbs slightly apart.
The pose is often
recommended for
loosening the muscles.

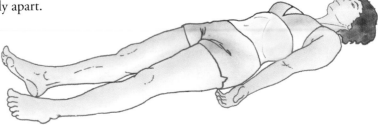

Indeed, when considered as a whole, the *conditions for equilibrium* are particularly easy to bring
about: the body rests on a surface of maximum support, and it is close to the ground. Therefore,
maintaining the pose does not require muscular contraction.

But, when observed *one joint at a time*, there are actually many contractions (small, but
consequential) which means that localized areas are not, on balance, relaxed. Two people can
experiment with this together, one person arranging and adjusting the other during the pose.

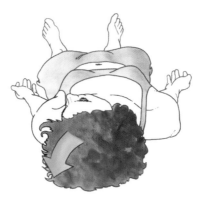

In the head and neck: In the
majority of cases the head is
not in balance, but rather
has a tendency to roll
towards one side or the other
(especially if the occiput is
rounded).

To keep the head from
falling, the musculature
of the neck contracts
in different places (this
contraction is frequently not
felt, as is generally the case
for the neck muscles, except
in cases of great fatigue, such
as during an illness).

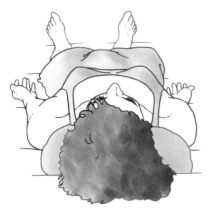

Your neck muscles will be more relaxed
if you place a wedge against each ear.

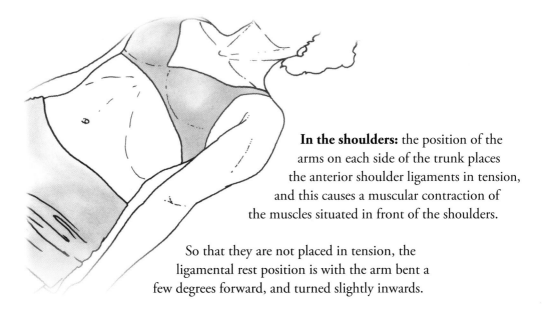

In the shoulders: the position of the arms on each side of the trunk places the anterior shoulder ligaments in tension, and this causes a muscular contraction of the muscles situated in front of the shoulders.

So that they are not placed in tension, the ligamental rest position is with the arm bent a few degrees forward, and turned slightly inwards.

Place a pillow under each arm to support this slight internal rotation. Or place the hands on the trunk with the elbows slightly bent.

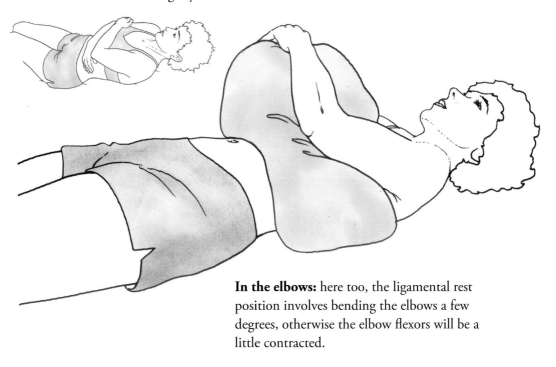

In the elbows: here too, the ligamental rest position involves bending the elbows a few degrees, otherwise the elbow flexors will be a little contracted.

Therefore, place a cushion under your wrists and hands.

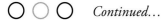 *Continued...*

In the hips and knees: so that there is no ligamental tension, the hips and knees must be slightly flexed. Otherwise, ligamental tension (moderate, but consequential) in the front of the hips and at the back of the knees causes contraction in the flexor muscles.

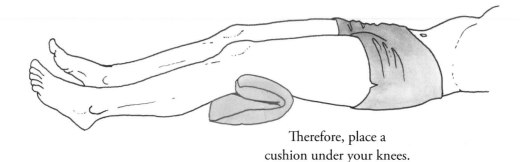

Therefore, place a cushion under your knees.

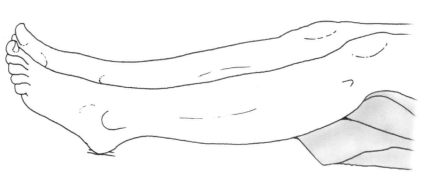

In the feet: without support, each foot falls into plantar flexion.

There is a need for support here, slight (the weight of the foot is reduced) but important: the anterior muscles of the leg are contracted.

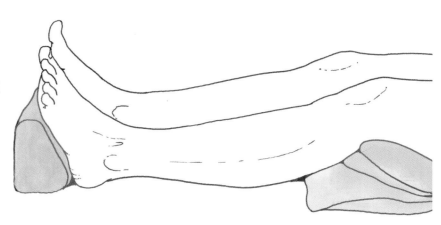

Your muscles will be more relaxed if you place a support under the sole of each foot.

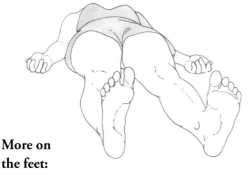

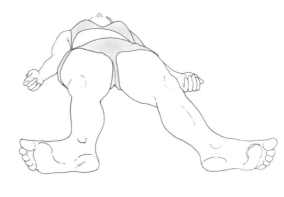

**More on
the feet:**
they fall outwards (which splays them a bit).
Higher up, this pulls the hips into external
rotation. But, seeing as the feet do not rest on
their outer edges when placed on the ground,
they are "off-supported" and this causes defi-
nite tension in the anterior hip ligaments.

So that the anterior hip ligaments
can relax completely, place a support
on the outer edge of each foot to
prevent them from falling into
external rotation.

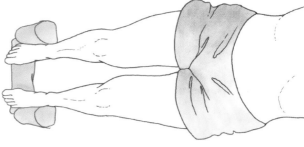

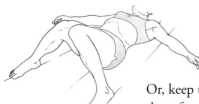

Or, keep the legs flexing internally to keep
them from both splaying and turning.

Conclusion: *Shavasana* is certainly a pose of *relief,* where the weight of the body does not have
to be borne, which makes it a pose of *general relief* for the main balance muscles. But, at the
level of each joint, the position brought about by the pose is not conducive to deep muscular
relaxation.

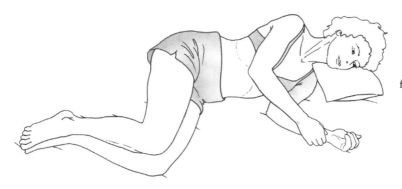

The optimal conditions
for muscular and articular
relaxation just described
can, rather, be brought
about by lying on one's
side, often called the
"recovery position."

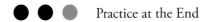 Practice at the End

Relax the deltoid muscles in
Sukhasana (Easy Pose)

In seated poses, we are often asked to place our relaxed arms on top of our lower limbs. In practice, how can we bring about this relaxation?

Here we will observe the *deltoid* muscle (AOM, p. 132), which is important to relax in order to free the deep components of the shoulder. We will start by describing certain structures of the joint.

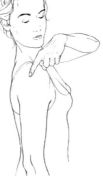

Looking over the shoulder, the acromion (1) forms a kind of "roof" above the upper part of the humerus.

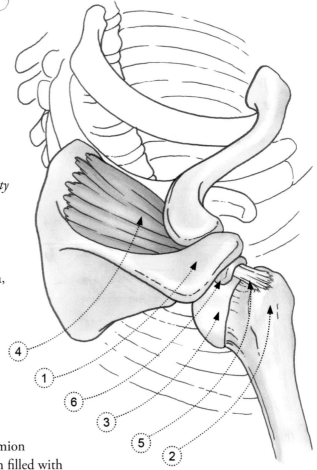

Above the humerus, the head of the humerus (3) articulates the *glenoid cavity* of the scapula, allowing the arm a great variety of movements. Several deep muscles surround the joint.

Among them, lodged above the scapula, the *supraspinatus* (4) is extended by a *tendon* (5) that passes under the acromion before attaching outside of the head of the humerus. It mobilizes the humerus (2), but often, its function is to hold it in place, suspended by its tendon.

To prevent it from chafing on the acromion during movement, a minuscule cushion filled with lubricating liquid, called the *synovial bursa*, is interposed between the tendon and the bone.

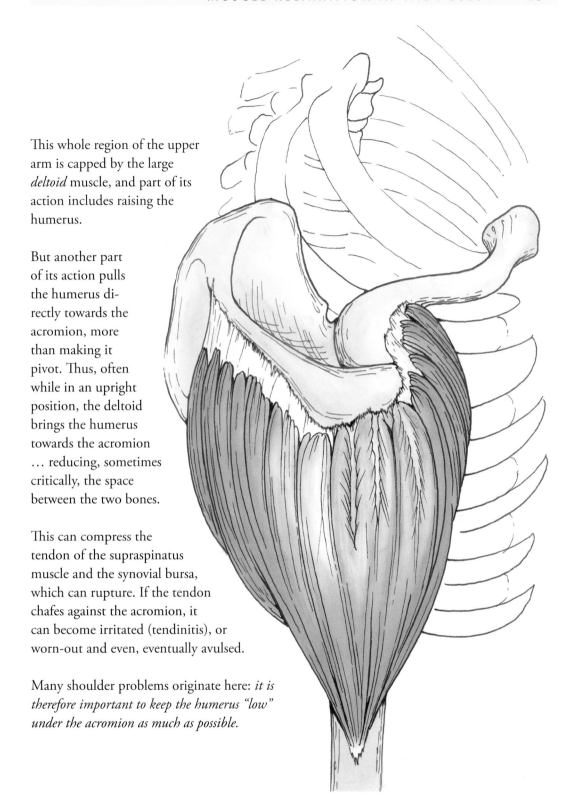

This whole region of the upper arm is capped by the large *deltoid* muscle, and part of its action includes raising the humerus.

But another part of its action pulls the humerus directly towards the acromion, more than making it pivot. Thus, often while in an upright position, the deltoid brings the humerus towards the acromion … reducing, sometimes critically, the space between the two bones.

This can compress the tendon of the supraspinatus muscle and the synovial bursa, which can rupture. If the tendon chafes against the acromion, it can become irritated (tendinitis), or worn-out and even, eventually avulsed.

Many shoulder problems originate here: *it is therefore important to keep the humerus "low" under the acromion as much as possible.*

For this, you can either lower it actively (see p. 202) or try to *relax* the deltoid.

○ ○ ○   *Continued…*

We can observe this relaxation of the deltoid in *Sukhasana*. Depending on how the arm and forearm are placed, you can either relax the shoulder muscles or, instead, contract them. Here are two of the many ways to place the arms.

1) While seated: the elbows fall into extension: if you position your upper limbs so that the upper part of the forearm is placed on your leg, the weight will cause your elbow to go into extension.

To prevent this extension from increasing, you must contract the muscles (the elbow flexors) in the front of your arm.

By proximity, this has a tendency to affect the neighboring muscle: the front of the deltoid.

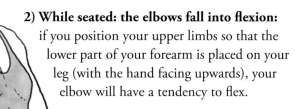

2) While seated: the elbows fall into flexion: if you position your upper limbs so that the lower part of your forearm is placed on your leg (with the hand facing upwards), your elbow will have a tendency to flex.

Therefore you must contract the muscles at the back of your arm (the triceps and the elbow extensor muscles) to prevent this flexion from increasing.

This has a tendency to affect the neighboring muscle, that is to say, the back of the deltoid.

In these two cases, you cannot relax your deltoid muscles, even if the instructions are to release the arms. But you can minimize the contraction. This is something to be vigilant about, particularly if the pose is held for a long time.

How? Try not to "squeeze" the upper arm under the acromion, and imagine instead that you are adding space to this area.

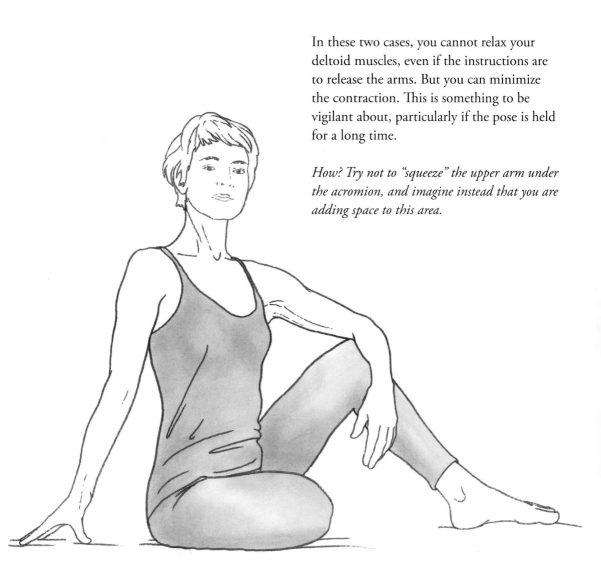

Supported forearm: you can also look for a method of arm placement that *allows the arm to be truly supported, in a position where it is neither flexed nor extended.* This is rather personal, and the choice of sitting position depends on the length of the thighs, the arms, and the range of motion in the hips. This may require orienting your forearm so that the hand is turned towards the ground.

Situation Analysis

Support the trunk for muscular relaxation in
Balasana (Child's Pose)

In this pose, the trunk flexes on itself and on the thighs. The head rests on the forehead, on the ground. *Depending on a few details, this either allows for or doesn't allow for muscular relaxation.*

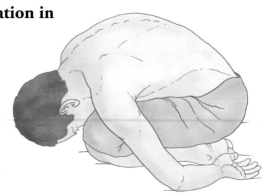

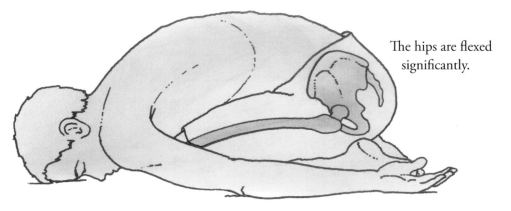

The hips are flexed significantly.

This is accentuated in certain variants of the pose, such as when the knees are slightly spread and the trunk is placed between the thighs.

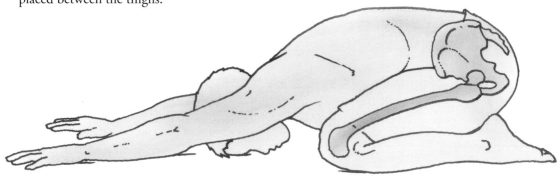

But the flexion can be limited (by posterior ligaments or muscles that are too short, but also, if one is overweight, by the stomach mass and the thighs meeting, or even by a broken bone in the front of the hip).

In these cases, the weight of the trunk cannot be placed on the thighs. The ligaments will tense and the muscles will not relax.

Sometimes a large, firm bolster is placed under the trunk. The effect of this support is two-fold:

• It *releases* the trunk. This allows the back muscles to relax.

• But also, it *diminishes* the range of flexion in the hip, and *allows a choice of range,* with all the consequences discussed above regarding the chosen tension of the posterior ligaments and the possibility of relaxing the muscles in this region.

Several options can be investigated:

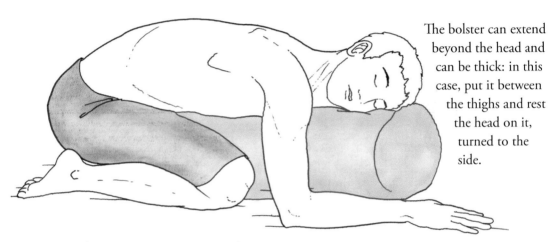

The bolster can extend beyond the head and can be thick: in this case, put it between the thighs and rest the head on it, turned to the side.

Warning: this can constrain the cervical vertebrae, since the rotation of the head reaches 90 degrees. For certain people, this can stretch the ligaments too much, without allowing the muscles to relax.

The bolster can also be placed only under the trunk: in this case, the knees are together and the bolster is placed on top of the knees.

Place the head on the bolster, resting on the chin.

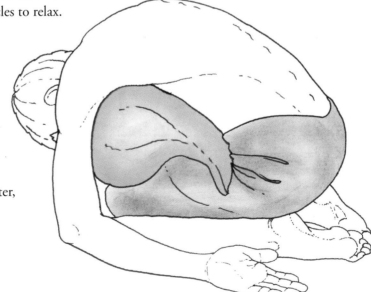

Situation Analysis

Relax the adductors in *Supta Baddha Konasana* (Supine Bound Angle Pose)

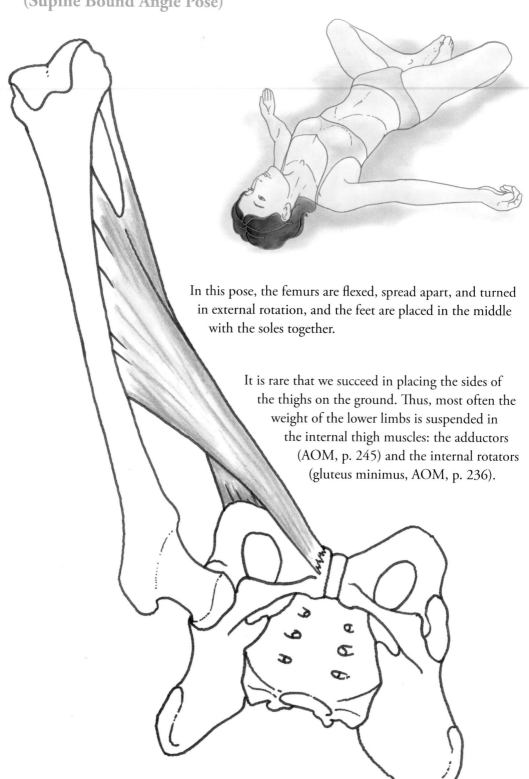

In this pose, the femurs are flexed, spread apart, and turned in external rotation, and the feet are placed in the middle with the soles together.

It is rare that we succeed in placing the sides of the thighs on the ground. Thus, most often the weight of the lower limbs is suspended in the internal thigh muscles: the adductors (AOM, p. 245) and the internal rotators (gluteus minimus, AOM, p. 236).

Several modifications can be proposed to allow
the hip muscles to relax and better extend.

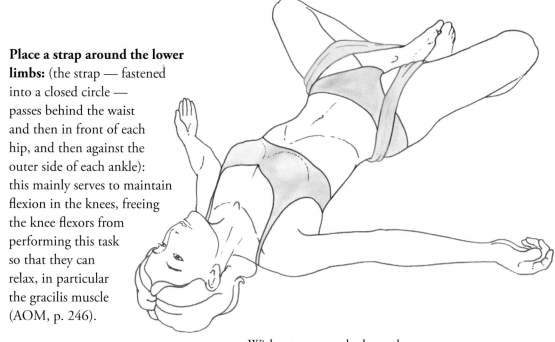

**Place a strap around the lower
limbs:** (the strap — fastened
into a closed circle —
passes behind the waist
and then in front of each
hip, and then against the
outer side of each ankle):
this mainly serves to maintain
flexion in the knees, freeing
the knee flexors from
performing this task
so that they can
relax, in particular
the gracilis muscle
(AOM, p. 246).

Without a strap, the knees have a
tendency to "stretch out" and cause
the legs to lengthen on the ground,
particularly if the ground or the
carpet is slippery.

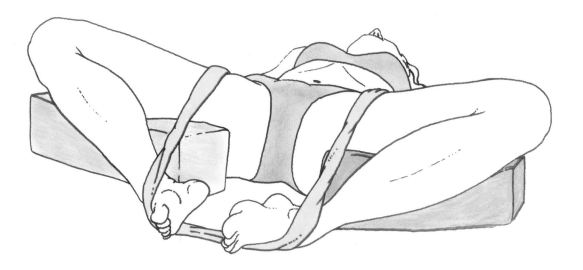

Place a block or a bolster under the thighs: this mainly serves to support the
weight of the thighs and the leg.

Continued...

Note: the range of motion in the two hips may not be symmetrical (this is usually the case).

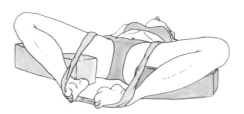

If you use supports that are the same height, there are two possible options:

• the thickness of the support may fit the more "open" hip (here the right hip).

This hip will be effectively sup-ported. But for the other hip, the height of the support does not allow the thigh or the leg to be placed on it, and so the muscles will not relax because they are contracted in order to hold this weight.

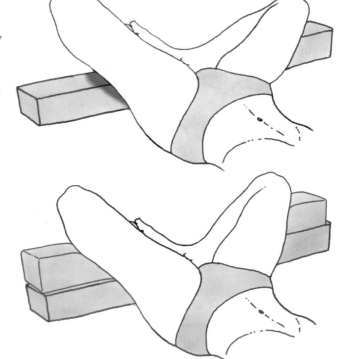

• or, the thickness of the support may fit the less "open" hip. Both hips will be supported. But the more open hip will be in a closed position. Its muscles will be — needlessly — held in the short position.

It is therefore preferable to use asymmetrical supports.

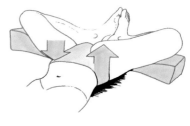

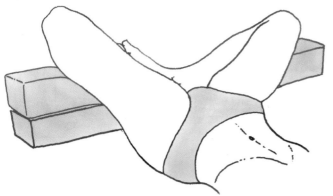

One solution often adopted by the practitioner without even realizing it is to position the pelvis asymmetrically in order to place each hip at an angle where it is supported correctly. But the bearing of the pelvis on the ground becomes asymmetrical (with more pressure on one buttock than the other), with all the consequences that this can have for the trunk.

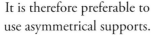

**Insert cushions under the head, the chest, and the upper part of the
waist:** this places the upper part of the trunk higher than the pelvis, and,
in the hip, returns it to flexion of the pelvis.

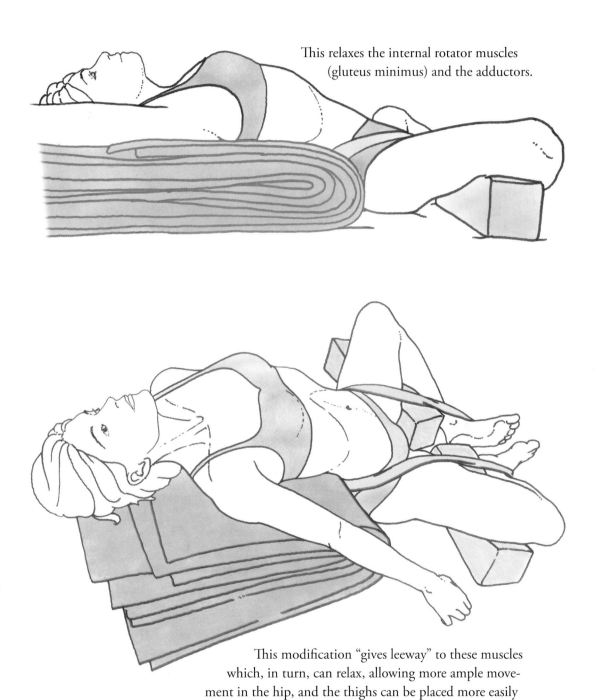

This relaxes the internal rotator muscles
(gluteus minimus) and the adductors.

This modification "gives leeway" to these muscles
which, in turn, can relax, allowing more ample movement in the hip, and the thighs can be placed more easily
on the ground or the side cushions.

Situation Analysis

Relax and contract on the correct side in
Ardha Chandrasana (Half-Moon Pose)

In this pose, each vertebra produces a lateral movement of lateral flexion from the vertebra below. This creates a curve, with a small concave side (the side towards which one bends), and a large convex side (opposite).

The curve is produced by the intervertebral joints. On either side of the vertebrae there is an area that is influenced by this lateral movement: the *intervertebral foramina* (AOM, p. 36).

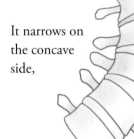

It narrows on the concave side,

and enlarges on the convex side.

The *spinal nerve* (in yellow in the illustration) passes through each intervertebral foramen. It is very close to the disc and is influenced by deformations in the disc during bending movements.

The weight of the trunk as a cantilever: in standing in ***Ardha Chandrasana*** (**Half-Moon Pose**), the head is not vertically symmetrical to the pelvis, but is offset to one side.

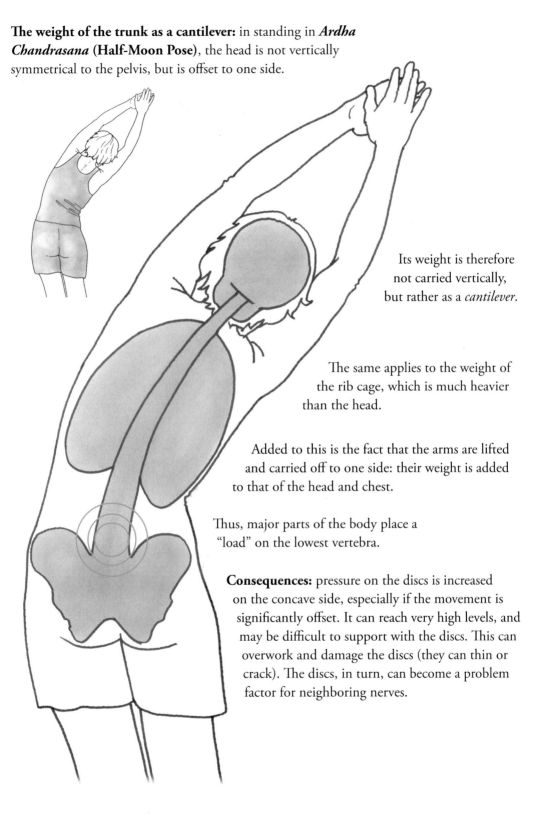

Its weight is therefore not carried vertically, but rather as a *cantilever*.

The same applies to the weight of the rib cage, which is much heavier than the head.

Added to this is the fact that the arms are lifted and carried off to one side: their weight is added to that of the head and chest.

Thus, major parts of the body place a "load" on the lowest vertebra.

Consequences: pressure on the discs is increased on the concave side, especially if the movement is significantly offset. It can reach very high levels, and may be difficult to support with the discs. This can overwork and damage the discs (they can thin or crack). The discs, in turn, can become a problem factor for neighboring nerves.

We can therefore see that during lateral flexion, this pressure must be moderated to protect both the discs and the nerves.

Continued…

To moderate the curve, it is necessary to contract the muscles on the convex side of the spine.

Note, however: if you bend, for example, to the right, — with the movement going towards the right — it is common to think that the muscles must also contract on the right (on the side towards which you lean). This is especially the case since we often "feel" the short side more clearly, as it is folded and tightened, and since the stretch is felt on the long side, this leads one to believe that the convex side must only stretch without any contraction.

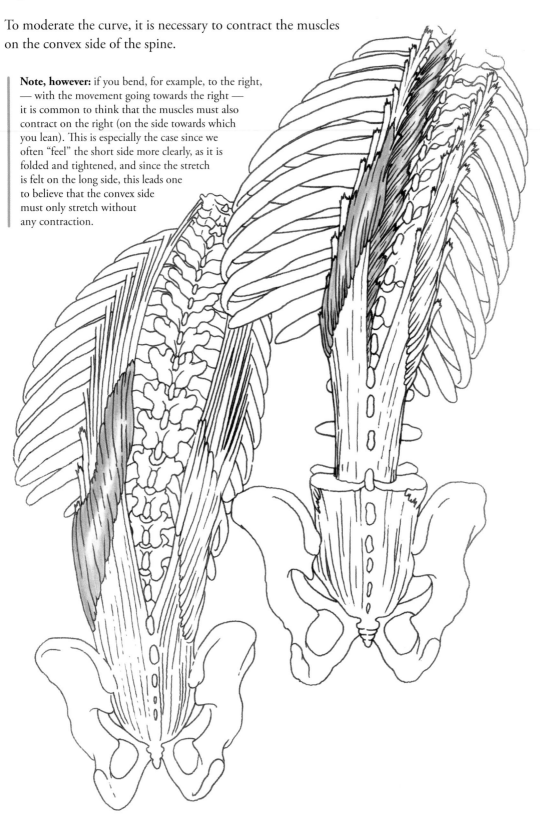

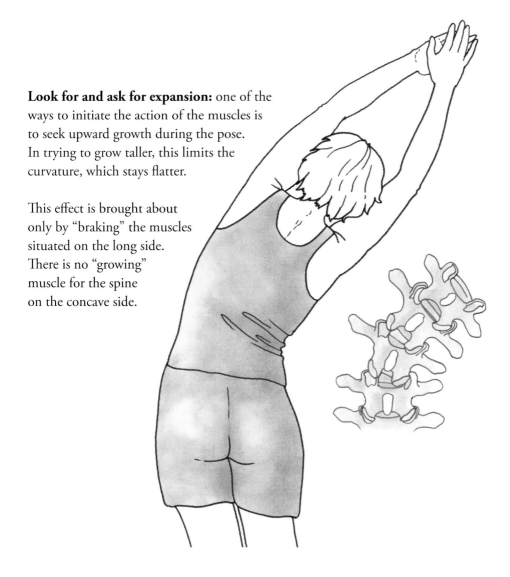

Look for and ask for expansion: one of the ways to initiate the action of the muscles is to seek upward growth during the pose. In trying to grow taller, this limits the curvature, which stays flatter.

This effect is brought about only by "braking" the muscles situated on the long side. There is no "growing" muscle for the spine on the concave side.

Mention muscle action rather than relaxation: when teaching this pose, it is important to say that we are trying to tone the long side. You can even touch the long side to feel the action of contraction.

Conversely, it is a mistake to call for relaxation of the long side to bring about this movement, since then the protection offered by these muscles would disappear. The only area where you can mention muscular relaxation is on the short side (concave side) of the curve.

This is found in the poses where the trunk is curved to one side:

Trikonasana **(Triangle Pose),**
Janusirasana **(Head-to-Knee Pose),**
Parighasana **(Gate Pose).**

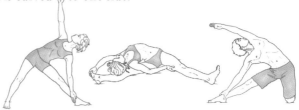

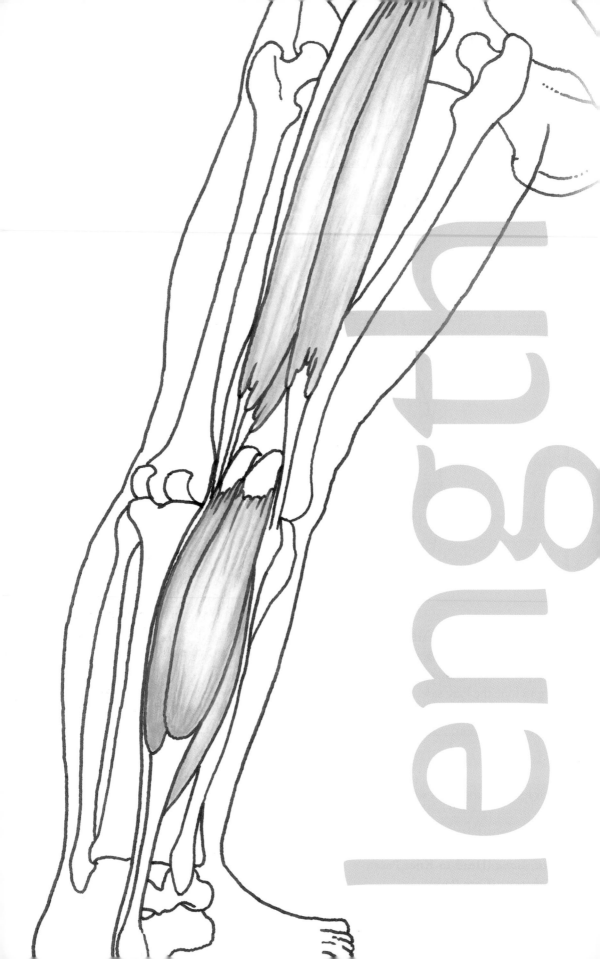

Muscle Length and the Poses

One of the characteristics of yoga is that it trains the body in positions that are not at all routine. What does the knee flexion in *Virasana* have in common with that which is needed in daily life, for example to sit in a chair or to go down the stairs?

Yoga explores the *ranges of movement* that can enhance the most common capacities. At the same time, practicing certain poses requires uncommon flexibility and, reciprocally, the stretches often soften the muscles involved. However, these ranges of movement are not always easy for the body: it is not always ready. There is a risk of hurting certain structures. Of all the tissues engaged in experiencing ranges of movement, the muscles are at the forefront. Almost all the poses require length in one or more muscles. It is this aspect that is explored in this chapter.

Observations on muscular length and muscle lengthening

A muscle that is never
stretched naturally tends
to shorten with time.

Muscle length varies from one person to another, and even for the same person it varies depending on the circumstances.

What stretches a muscle is *the inverse movement of its action.*

For example, to stretch the gluteus maximus, which is a hip extensor,

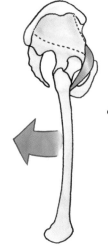

there must be hip flexion.

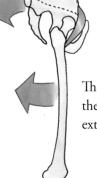

The stretching movement can be carried out by one or the other of the bones attached to the muscle: for the iliacus muscle, which is a hip flexor, the stretching movement can be brought about by the femur (femur extension)

or by the pelvis (extension of the pelvis).

The movement can also be carried out by the two bones at once (simultaneous femur extension and extension of the pelvis).

Stretching a biarticular muscle

If the muscle is attached to three bones, stretching it requires the inverse of its action at the two joints that it crosses.

For example, the rectus femoris muscle of the thigh is attached on top to the iliacus bone, and to the tibia on the bottom.

It crosses both the hip and the knee. In order for it to stretch, both hip extension and knee flexion are required simultaneously. If only one of these two movements is performed, the muscle will not stretch.

State of activity of a stretched muscle

A muscle undergoing this stretching movement can either be passive (that is, a muscle stretch proper) or active (the muscle contracts, but the inverse movement is taking place; that is, an eccentric contraction. For more on this, see p. 24).

A muscle is not stretched by its own action. It is stretched by actions produced from forces external to it, which can be quite varied.

For example, for the squat in *Malasana* (Garland pose), it is gravity that brings about the hip flexion, and the gluteus maximus is stretched by this movement.

For the elbow flexion in *Gomukhasana* (Cow Face Pose), it is the traction of the opposite hand that creates the flexion that stretches the extensor muscle of the elbow (the triceps).

For *Paschimmottanasana* (Seated Forward Bend), it is gravity added to the traction of the hands that creates the forward movement of the trunk.

Thus, for these three examples, the expression "the buttock stretches" or "the triceps stretch" is an image often used in the language of physical technique, but does not correspond to reality.

Stretching red muscle

In the contractile parts of the muscle mass, stretching produces a shifting and distancing of actin and myosin filaments. As seen on p. 14, this does not exclude contraction.

The diagram shows that the number of myosin heads in contact with actin filaments decreases. The effect is a reduction in contractile force.

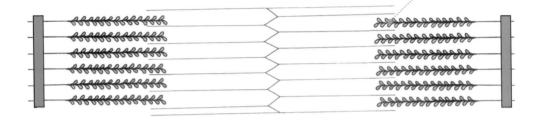

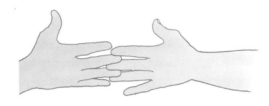

Titin description (see also p. 14).

Titin is a giant protein that connects the Z line to the A line. It is represented here as a spring, which, for the simplicity of the drawing, links the myosin to line Z.

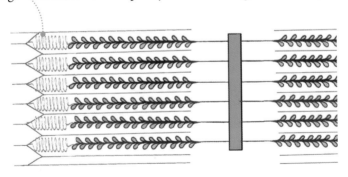

It plays an important role in maintaining the structure of sarcomere, and contributes to its elasticity.

When a muscular fiber is stretched, the titin is gradually placed in tension. This has the effect of unfolding the molecular chains and placing them in tension.

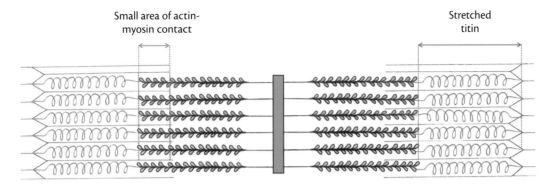

Small area of actin-myosin contact

Stretched titin

These will act like a spring and exert an elastic return force. Through its form and composition, titin contributes to making muscle fiber a passive tensor when it is stretched beyond its resting length.

During stretching, muscle force is thus the result of two components whose importance varies according to the intensity of stretching:

- in low-intensity stretching, it is the actin-myosin coupling that predominates
- in high-intensity stretching, it is the elastic return of the titin.

Stretching white muscle

In the aponeuroses, elongation places in tension the collagen fibers that make up a part of the enveloping connective tissue. They tend to align more closely.

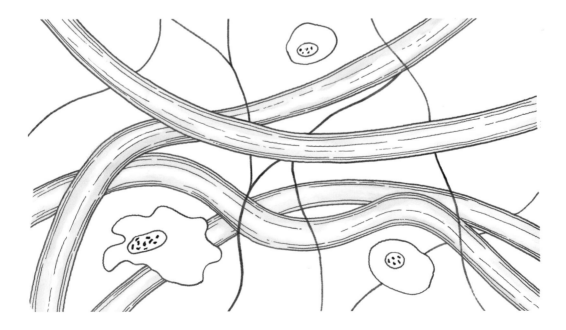

THE FOLLOWING PAGES will present, through cases involving yoga poses, the *principal muscles that are stretched in yoga*. Two scenarios are presented:

- Can the pose be taken straight away in order to stretch the muscle? If so, what are the benefits of this stretch?

- Is it necessary for the muscle to be stretched prior to practicing the pose correctly? If so, stretching exercises are proposed.

Note   Each themed explanation sheet presents just one example, and not the entirety:

- For each pose, one single muscle or muscular group is presented in its stretching state. But it is obvious that this muscle is not the only one being stretched in the pose.

- Furthermore, the pose presented is not the only one in yoga that stretches this muscle. Each explanation sheet therefore indicates several other poses that stretch the same muscle.

14 Themed Explanation Sheets: Poses Discussed

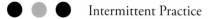

Long hamstring muscles
in *Dandasana* (Staff Pose)

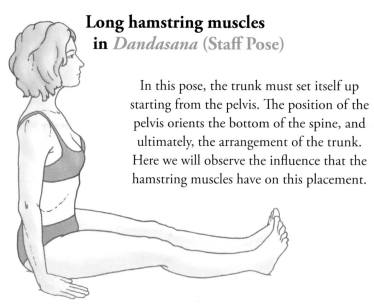

In this pose, the trunk must set itself up starting from the pelvis. The position of the pelvis orients the bottom of the spine, and ultimately, the arrangement of the trunk. Here we will observe the influence that the hamstring muscles have on this placement.

Perform and observe some pelvic movements: place yourself in *Vajrasana* **(Thunderbolt or Diamond Pose)**, or sit on a very low seat so that the hips are bent 90 degrees and the knees are also bent.

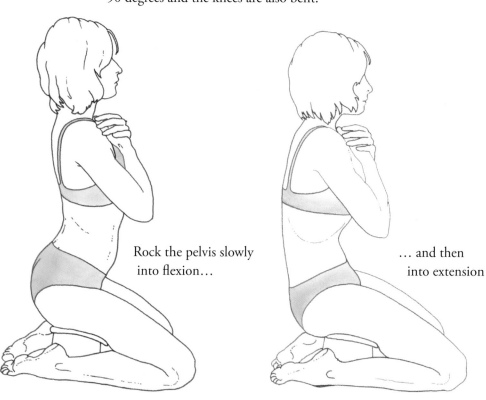

Rock the pelvis slowly into flexion…

… and then into extension

Flexion of the pelvis and the curve of the waist: with the flat of your hand, trace the waist area. Locate the lumbar vertebrae, which form a slight hollow in back (lordosis). This is the natural curvature of the lumbar region. When the pelvis is flexed, the lumbar spine still forms this curve higher up.

Lower the hand a little and feel the form of the sacrum, bulging slightly behind.

Slide your hand up and down several times to feel the *double curve:* below, the bulging sacrum and above, the slightly-hollowed waist area.

Extension of the pelvis and removal of the curve: go into extension of the pelvis. Pass the hand over the back: feel how the lumbar hollow has disappeared.

Repeat the exercise, in both ways, to feel how the movement of the pelvis and the lumbar spine are linked. Then, place your pelvis clearly in flexion.

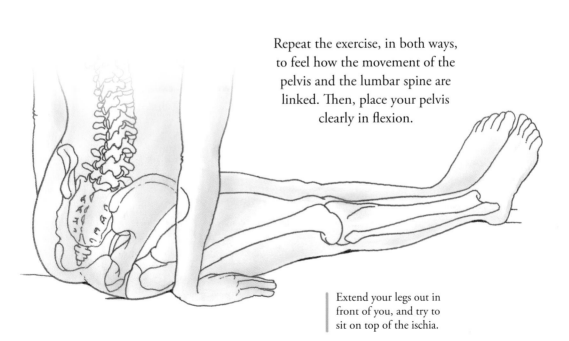

Extend your legs out in front of you, and try to sit on top of the ischia.

○ ○ ○   *Continued…*

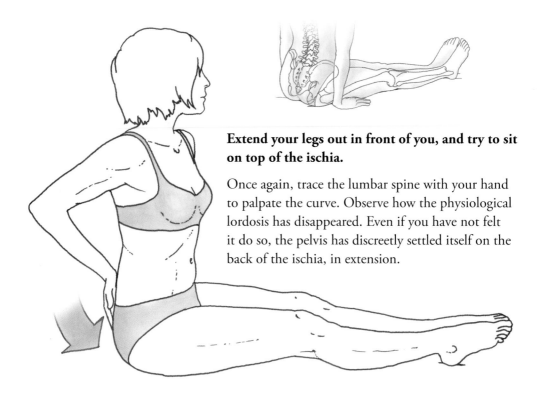

Extend your legs out in front of you, and try to sit on top of the ischia.

Once again, trace the lumbar spine with your hand to palpate the curve. Observe how the physiological lordosis has disappeared. Even if you have not felt it do so, the pelvis has discreetly settled itself on the back of the ischia, in extension.

This extension of the pelvis is not chosen — in the way that you just experimented with — but rather is caused by placing the hamstring muscles in tension (AOM, p. 242).

These muscles are placed in tension each time we combine hip flexion with knee extension. They pull their attachments up, and the ischia pull the whole pelvis into extension.

Often too short, the hamstring muscles "make the rules" for the pelvis and place it in extension when we sit with our legs extended.

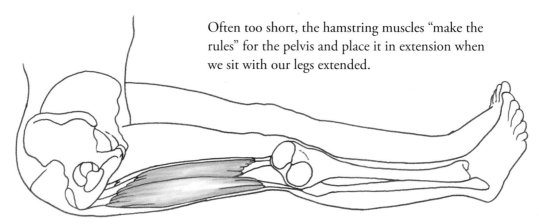

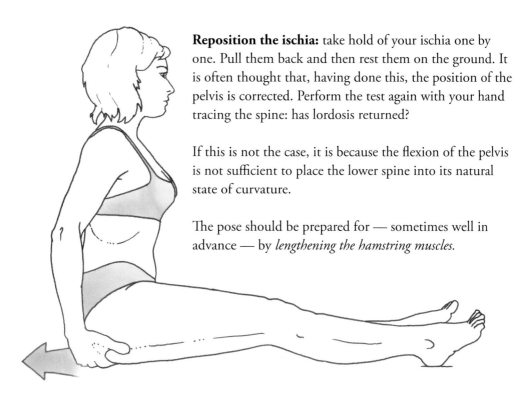

Reposition the ischia: take hold of your ischia one by one. Pull them back and then rest them on the ground. It is often thought that, having done this, the position of the pelvis is corrected. Perform the test again with your hand tracing the spine: has lordosis returned?

If this is not the case, it is because the flexion of the pelvis is not sufficient to place the lower spine into its natural state of curvature.

The pose should be prepared for — sometimes well in advance — by *lengthening the hamstring muscles.*

Elevate your pelvis: in the meantime, it is advisable to practice ***Dandasana*** by placing yourself on one (or several) blocks made of hard foam, which will diminish the angle of flexion in your hips, thus allowing the hamstrings to be less tensed. Your pelvis will become freer again, and your lumbar spine too. This modification helps protect your spine when the hamstrings are not sufficiently long.

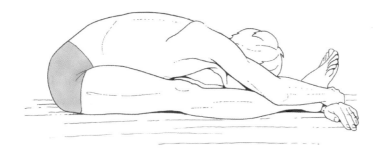

Being able to move the ischia back in ***Dandasana*** is essential for practicing another pose: ***Paschimottanasana*** **(Seated Forward Bend)** (see p. 116).

Stretching the hamstring muscles

Protect the spine: the hamstrings are powerful muscles that are often short. They must be lengthened in a position where the pelvis and the vertebrae are not at risk of being pulled, especially when "loaded."

(use a long sash or strap)

The best method is for you to stretch out on your back, with the hips, knees and ankles bent, and the feet flat. The ground will act as an *alignment guardian* that protects your back. Raise one leg, foot towards the ceiling.

Position the leg: pass the strap or sash under the foot and loop it around once to fix it in place. Do not place the strap too far forward (so as to exclude the gastrocnemius muscle from the stretch), but rather at the instep. Bring the leg up to vertical.

Very important: if necessary, keep the knee bent. Then, alternate the following three exercises, initially performing them separately.

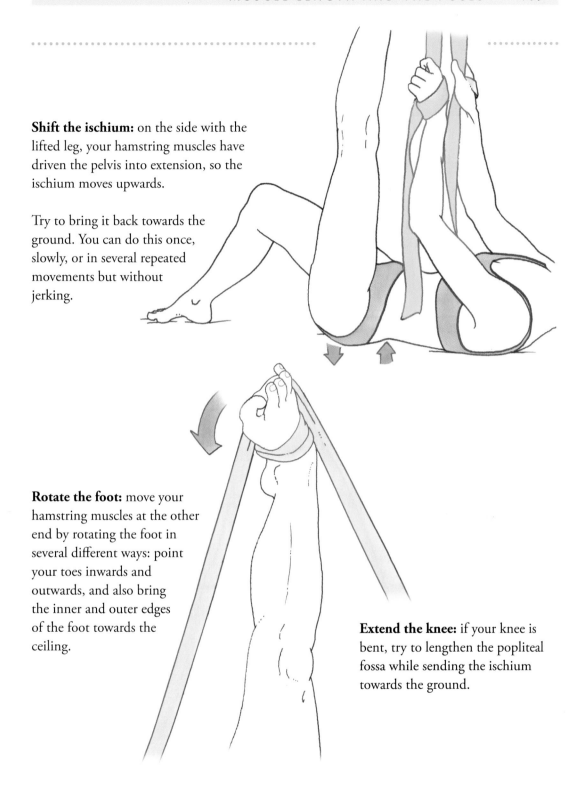

Shift the ischium: on the side with the lifted leg, your hamstring muscles have driven the pelvis into extension, so the ischium moves upwards.

Try to bring it back towards the ground. You can do this once, slowly, or in several repeated movements but without jerking.

Rotate the foot: move your hamstring muscles at the other end by rotating the foot in several different ways: point your toes inwards and outwards, and also bring the inner and outer edges of the foot towards the ceiling.

Extend the knee: if your knee is bent, try to lengthen the popliteal fossa while sending the ischium towards the ground.

For people with "resistant" hamstring muscles, this work should be repeated regularly, possibly preceded by a massage of the back of the thigh.

Above all, do not practice poses with flexed hips and straight legs without having prepared these muscles first.

Situation Analysis

Long hamstring muscles and/or gastrocnemius muscles in
Adho Mukha Svanasana (Downward-Facing Dog Pose)

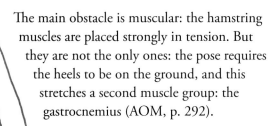

In this pose, you are on all fours and create a triangle with the pelvis as the highest point. In order for the entire spine to experience well-aligned decompression, the pelvis should be oriented with the "ischia towards the ceiling." But they don't always move freely.

The main obstacle is muscular: the hamstring muscles are placed strongly in tension. But they are not the only ones: the pose requires the heels to be on the ground, and this stretches a second muscle group: the gastrocnemius (AOM, p. 292).

The gastrocnemius muscle is part of the triceps surae muscle of the calf. On top it is attached to the femur, and on the bottom to the Achilles tendon on the calcaneus (the heel bone). It therefore crosses the knee and the ankle.

The gastrocnemius muscle is stretched when you simultaneously "flex" the foot while extending the knee. In **Adho Mukha Svanasana** they are placed strongly in tension, and if they are too short, they tend to either bend the knee(s) or raise the heel(s).

It is not always possible for a beginner to fully achieve the correct pose form with regard to two muscle groups: the hamstring muscles and the gastrocnemius muscles. We can therefore observe — and suggest — two modifications:

If the gastrocnemius muscles are short (particularly in the case of people who wear high-heeled shoes) and for whom the hamstring muscles are sufficiently long: it is easier, in this case, to *place the hands closer to the feet.*

This requires more hip flexion, but less range of motion in the ankle.

If the hamstring muscles are short, and the gastrocnemius muscles are long: the person will have a limit to their hip flexion.

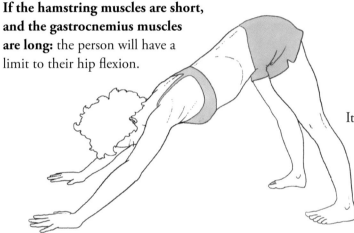

It is easier, in this case, to place the hands farther from the feet. This requires less hip flexion, and more flexion in the ankle.

If both muscles are short, three modifications are suggested:

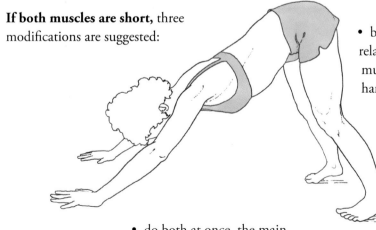

• bend the knees a little: this relaxes both the *gastrocnemius* muscles as well as the hamstring muscles,

• let the heels leave the ground: this decreases the ankle flexion and relaxes the *gastrocnemius* muscles,

• do both at once, the main point in **Adho Mukha Svanasana** being to ensure that the pelvis is oriented "ischia upwards."

Stretching the triceps surae (gastrocnemius and soleus muscles)

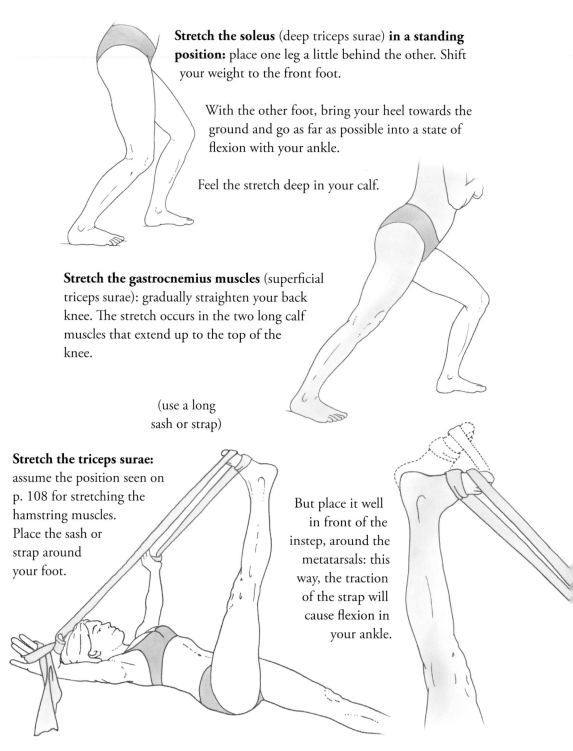

Stretch the soleus (deep triceps surae) **in a standing position:** place one leg a little behind the other. Shift your weight to the front foot.

With the other foot, bring your heel towards the ground and go as far as possible into a state of flexion with your ankle.

Feel the stretch deep in your calf.

Stretch the gastrocnemius muscles (superficial triceps surae): gradually straighten your back knee. The stretch occurs in the two long calf muscles that extend up to the top of the knee.

(use a long sash or strap)

Stretch the triceps surae: assume the position seen on p. 108 for stretching the hamstring muscles. Place the sash or strap around your foot.

But place it well in front of the instep, around the metatarsals: this way, the traction of the strap will cause flexion in your ankle.

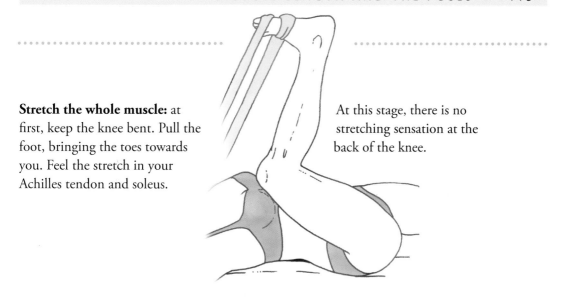

Stretch the whole muscle: at first, keep the knee bent. Pull the foot, bringing the toes towards you. Feel the stretch in your Achilles tendon and soleus.

At this stage, there is no stretching sensation at the back of the knee.

Rotate the foot: using the strap, turn your foot so that your toes point inwards and outwards, and also bring the inner and outer edges of the foot towards the ceiling.

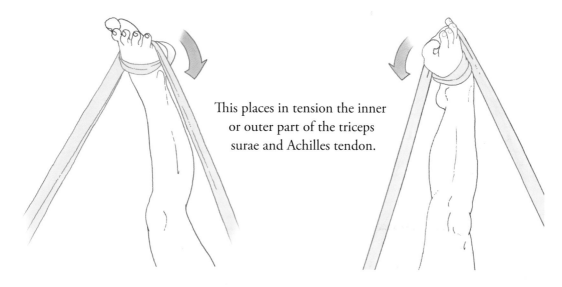

This places in tension the inner or outer part of the triceps surae and Achilles tendon.

Stretch the gastrocnemius: first bend the other leg, knee towards the stomach, to roll the pelvis into extension. Then return to the leg with the strap. Keeping the ankle flexed, gradually lengthen the knee: the calf stretch will extend to the popliteal fossa behind the knee, stretching the upper part of the gastrocnemius.

Stretch the entire posterior muscle chain of the lower limb: take the leg that was bent towards your stomach and lay it out on the ground: your pelvis will return to flexion. Repeat the previous stretch, but now, both your hamstring muscles as well as your triceps surae will be lengthened.

● ● ●   Intermittent Practice

Long gluteus maximus muscles as a result of *Malasana* (Garland Pose)

In this pose, you sit squatting with the trunk flexed and resting on the thighs, knees bent.

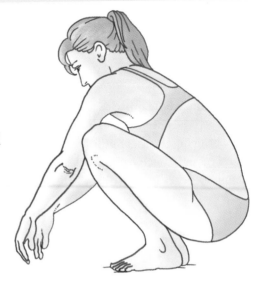

The weight of the trunk is placed on the front of the thighs, and the arms are carried somewhat forward.

At the hip, this pose produces *more flexion* than the two preceding poses (and the following one). Why?

Because with the knees bent, the hamstring muscles are not placed in tension, and do not limit the flexion in the hips, which can go farther into flexion (and even as far as is possible).

The flexion is so complete because the weight of the body rotates the pelvis.

This maximal hip flexion causes the gluteus maximus muscle to stretch (AOM, p. 249).

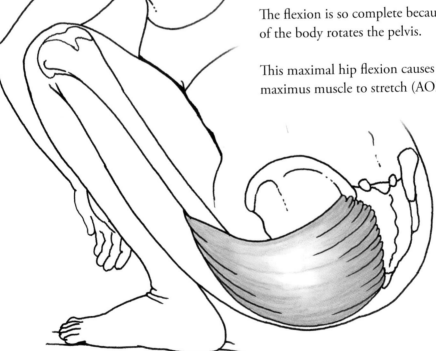

This is relevant to all the poses where length in the gluteus maximus is required. In particular, the poses in the *Padmasana* (**Lotus Pose**) series require flexibility of the gluteus maximus for the component involving movement of the flexed hip.

Actively flex the hip: lying on your back with your legs outstretched, bring one bent knee towards your chest.

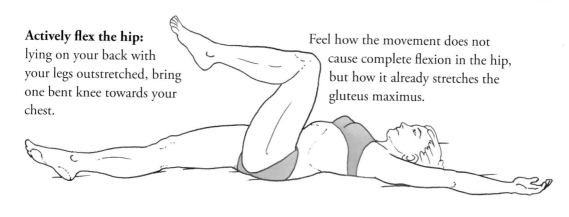

Feel how the movement does not cause complete flexion in the hip, but how it already stretches the gluteus maximus.

Passively flex the hip: now take the knee between your clasped hands and bend your elbows so that the knee presses firmly towards your stomach.

Feel how here, you are causing complete flexion of the hip, and how your gluteus maximus is completely stretched.

Position the pelvis: place a lift (such as a rolled-up towel) under the lower part of the waist. This will keep your pelvis slightly flexed.

Next, resume the preceding movement with the knees held in your hands (this is **Pavanamuktasana** or **Wind-Relieving Pose**).

Your gluteus maximus will encounter a greater stretch owing to the lift, since your pelvis can no longer compensate by going into extension.

Other poses that stretch the gluteus maximus: *Balasana* (**Child's Pose**), *Pavanamuktasana* (**Wind-Relieving Pose**), and *Anjaneyasana* (**Crescent Lunge on the Knee**) on the side where the hip is flexed.

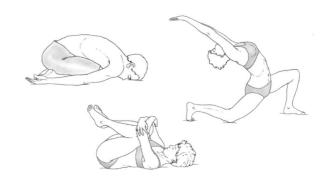

● ● ● Intermittent Practice

A long Latissimus dorsi muscle in *Paschimottanasana* (Seated Forward Bend)

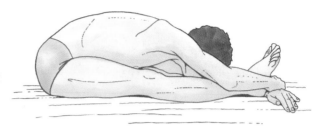

In this pose, you sit on the ground with the knees stretched out in front. The head, the trunk, and the arms are brought forward. Ideally, the entire movement *originates in the hip joints*: the pelvis pivots towards flexion, orienting the entire lumbar spine towards the front.

Thus, there is lots of movement in the pelvis and a small amount of flexion in the spine, which lengthens by settling onto the thighs rather than bending by itself.

Then it will be possible to bring about — without danger to the discs or nerves — what the pose is intended for: *stretching the entirety of the back of the body*, and particularly the widest contractile layer of the back: the latissimus dorsi muscle (AOM, p. 131).

For this, it is crucial that the hamstring muscles be long enough to allow the pelvis the freedom to roll towards the front as much as possible. (This means that at a minimum — before assuming this pose — you must be able to place yourself on the front of the ischia in *Dandasana,* shown on p. 107).*

This muscle is spread like a large fan from the pelvis to the sides, where it meets the arms.

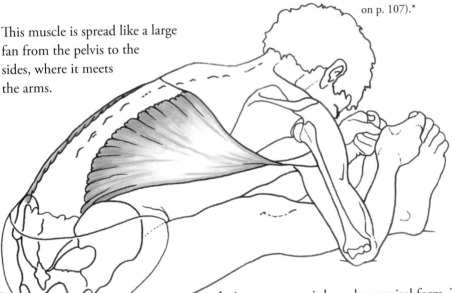

In its upper part it has a large spiral form. To stretch it, you must simultaneously bend the entire trunk into an elongated curve, while also bringing the arms far beyond the head. It is necessary to understand something regarding the position of the lumbar. Two exercises for this purpose are shown on the next page.

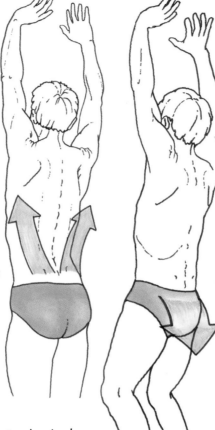

Stretch the latissimus dorsi muscle "from above": while standing, raise your arms to their maximum height. As they rise, the arm position stretches the upper part of the latissimus dorsi muscle. But, lower down, the lumbar region tends to hollow out, since the latissimus dorsi — its upper part placed in tension — pulls on its insertion in the pelvis.

Stretch the latissimus dorsi muscle "from below": keeping the same position, now move the pelvis into extension: feel how the lower part of the latissimus dorsi has elongated, stretching the whole muscle.

In *Paschimottanasana* it is the tension in the hamstring muscles that prevents the lumbar vertebrae from hollowing out. The back extended in long flexion and the arms carried far in front together bring about the complete stretch of the latissimus dorsi muscle.

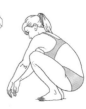

* If the hamstring muscles lack length, the pelvis will be unable to tilt and it will be the trunk that creates the bend as a great cantilever (because it cannot rest on the thighs). The pose can then cause lumbago and sciatica.

Therefore, if your hamstring muscles are still too short, it is best to stretch the latissimus dorsi muscle by hanging from a bar.

Other poses that stretch the latissimus dorsi muscle: *Uttanasana* (**Standing Forward Bend**), *Halasana* (**Plough Pose**) and *Malasana* (**Garland Pose**).

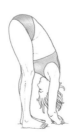
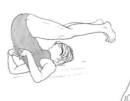

Intermittent Practice

A long trapezius muscle in
Halasana (Plough Pose)

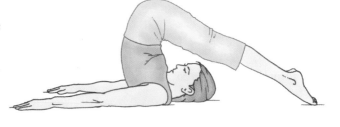

In this pose, the legs curl towards the trunk while you lie on your back, causing the trunk to bend. The feet pass behind the head and can rest on the ground.

There are many variations which will lengthen the different parts of the trapezius muscle to varying extents.

The trapezius is one of the largest muscle layers in the body; moreover, some segments are oriented from top to bottom, others from side to side, and others even from front to back (in the segment that attaches to the clavicles).

Few movements or poses stretch it completely.

You can feel and understand this through a simple preliminary exercise. Place yourself in a standing position, feet parallel and neck straight.

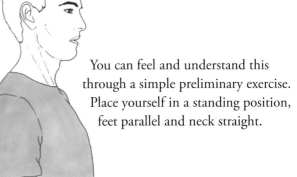

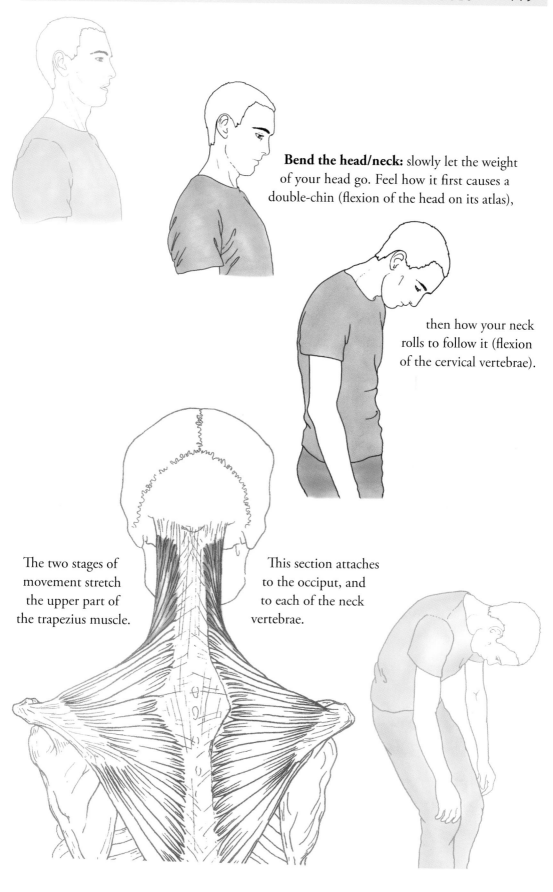

Bend the head/neck: slowly let the weight of your head go. Feel how it first causes a double-chin (flexion of the head on its atlas),

then how your neck rolls to follow it (flexion of the cervical vertebrae).

The two stages of movement stretch the upper part of the trapezius muscle.

This section attaches to the occiput, and to each of the neck vertebrae.

○ ○ ○   *Continued...*

Spread the scapulae: let the movement continue. Feel how the weight of the arms now pulls the shoulders, which move laterally away from the spinal column.

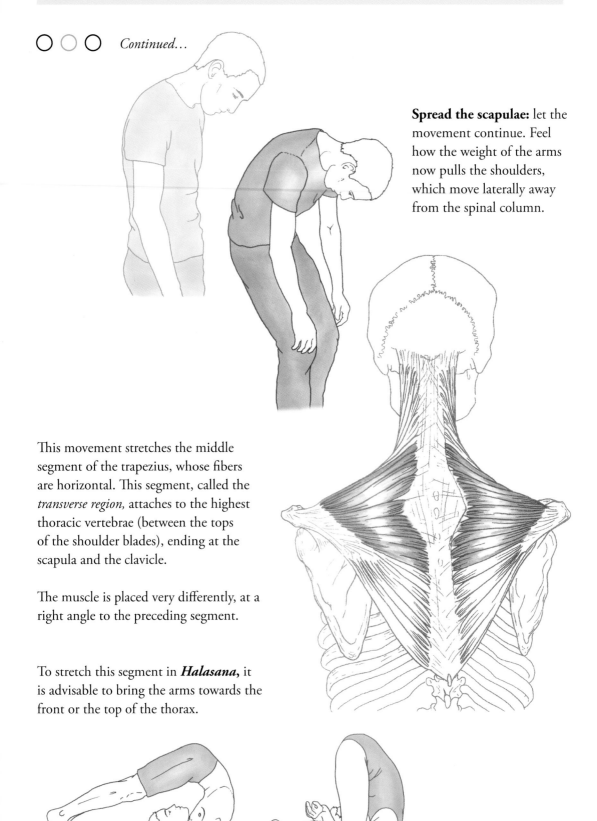

This movement stretches the middle segment of the trapezius, whose fibers are horizontal. This segment, called the *transverse region,* attaches to the highest thoracic vertebrae (between the tops of the shoulder blades), ending at the scapula and the clavicle.

The muscle is placed very differently, at a right angle to the preceding segment.

To stretch this segment in **Halasana,** it is advisable to bring the arms towards the front or the top of the thorax.

Bend the trunk: the movement now extends by rolling the thoracic vertebrae one over the other, one by one. Here, it is the lower part of the muscle that is stretched.

At this point, the trapezius attaches to the innermost part of the scapula to join the vertebrae at T12, forming a tip that covers part of the latissimus dorsi.

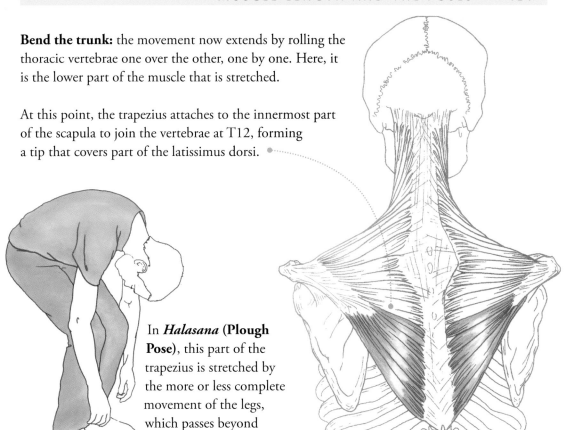

In *Halasana* (**Plough Pose**), this part of the trapezius is stretched by the more or less complete movement of the legs, which passes beyond the trunk.

The stretch is extended by that of the latissimus dorsi.

Bend the trunk "from below": now bring the trunk so that it is completely bent over the legs in triple flexion (the hips, the knees, and the ankles). The strong hip flexion pulls the pelvis into extension, which stretches the trapezius even more completely.

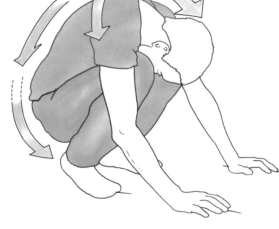

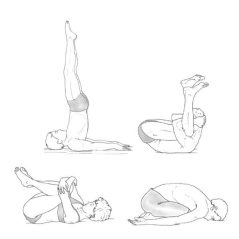

This can be found in *Sarvangasana* (**Shoulder-stand**) for the upper trapezius, *Ananda Balasana* (**Happy Baby Pose**) for the transverse trapezius, and in *Balasana* (**Child's Pose**) or **Extended Child's Pose** for the lower part of the trapezius.

Intermittent Practice

A long psoas muscle in *Anjaneyasana* (Crescent Lunge on the Knee)

In this pose, the arms are raised to the maximum in front, a movement that is extended with an extension of the whole spine.

The lower body must stabilize the pelvis in order to provide a solid base for this launch. This will stretch the psoas muscle (AOM, p. 234).

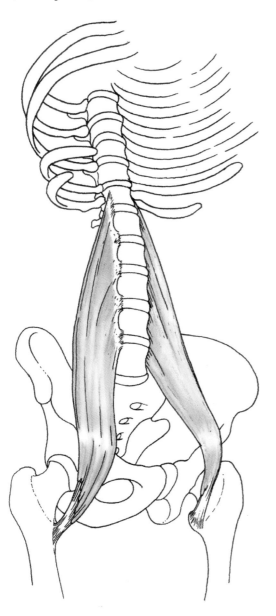

Set up the base: you can prepare the pose by starting in the so-called called "proposal position" where the supporting knee is not drawn back behind the trunk.

Observe how the pelvis tends to turn in two ways:

• one, it retracts and rises on the side of the back leg (one buttock is farther back and higher than the other);

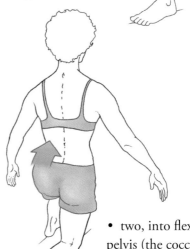

• two, into flexion of the pelvis (the coccyx tends to point backwards).

Move the back leg farther back: next, set up the bottom of the pose by moving the supporting leg back. Thus, the two movements that turn the pelvis increase strongly. They are the consequence of insufficient range of extension at the front of the hip.

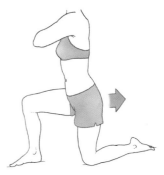

The psoas muscle is one of the obstacles preventing the femur from moving back and the pelvis from staying "neutral."

This deep muscle attaches, on top, to the lumbar vertebrae, then descends by curving in front of the pelvis (on the pubis) before heading back again and attaching itself to the lesser trochanter.

In *Anjaneyasana,* the psoas is placed in tension along the whole of its trajectory: it is stretched simultaneously by the extension of the spine and by the extension of the hip.

It tries to compensate by pushing the pubis back (which causes the first rotation seen above) and also by pushing it down (which creates flexion of the pelvis). It does not act through direct traction of the bones, but instead pushes the bones in the places where it curves over them.

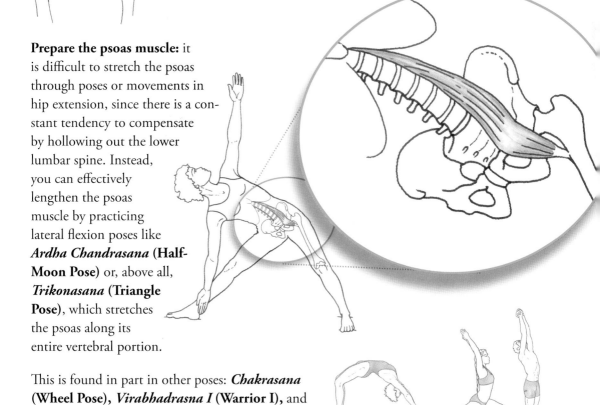

Prepare the psoas muscle: it is difficult to stretch the psoas through poses or movements in hip extension, since there is a constant tendency to compensate by hollowing out the lower lumbar spine. Instead, you can effectively lengthen the psoas muscle by practicing lateral flexion poses like ***Ardha Chandrasana* (Half-Moon Pose)** or, above all, ***Trikonasana* (Triangle Pose)**, which stretches the psoas along its entire vertebral portion.

This is found in part in other poses: ***Chakrasana* (Wheel Pose), *Virabhadrasna I* (Warrior I),** and the first movement in ***Surya Namaskara* (Sun Salutation)**.

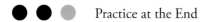

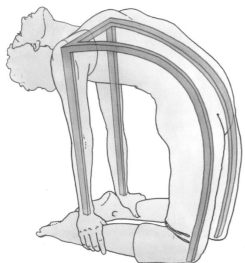

Long rectus femoris muscles
in *Ustrasana* (Camel Pose)

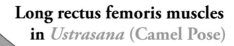

In this pose, the spine adopts a movement of extension. However, mobility between the vertebrae is not uniform along the spine: certain joints move only slightly, while others are highly mobile.

The lowest joint is called the *lumbosacral joint* or L5/S1 and is highly mobile in extension. In fact, that is the position it is in when we assume the pose. The intervertebral disc becomes distorted: it pinches together in back and stretches out a little in front.

In principle, a disk can support this, except in two cases: if there is a lot of pressure, or if the movement involves great range of motion in one single joint. And, above all, if these two situations coincide.

In *Ustrasana*, the range of extension is predominantly at L5/S1. What about pressure? Here, so that the weight of the trunk is not applied to the lower part of the spine, you must lean on your hands, which rest on your heels.

But, in order to do so, the hands must be able to reach the feet ... which requires sufficient range of extension in the spine. The amount of pressure and the range of motion are therefore linked.

In order to go back, bring the hands in contact with the feet. There are two other areas that must be brought into extension: the two hips. Their range of extension is usually reduced due to anatomical features found in front of the joint. Of these, we will observe the rectus femoris muscle (AOM, p. 238)

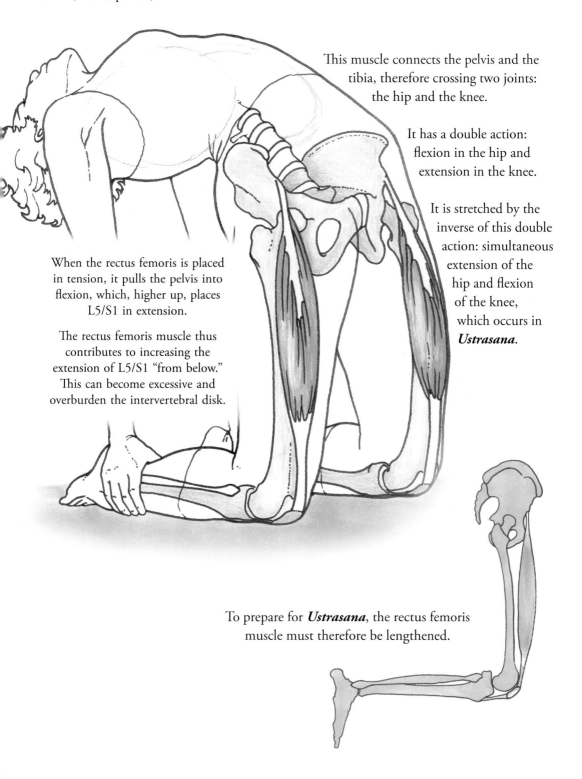

This muscle connects the pelvis and the tibia, therefore crossing two joints: the hip and the knee.

It has a double action: flexion in the hip and extension in the knee.

It is stretched by the inverse of this double action: simultaneous extension of the hip and flexion of the knee, which occurs in *Ustrasana*.

When the rectus femoris is placed in tension, it pulls the pelvis into flexion, which, higher up, places L5/S1 in extension.

The rectus femoris muscle thus contributes to increasing the extension of L5/S1 "from below." This can become excessive and overburden the intervertebral disk.

To prepare for *Ustrasana*, the rectus femoris muscle must therefore be lengthened.

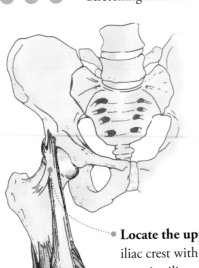

Stretching the rectus femoris muscle

For this exercise, use a very small cushion or lift. This can be a folded handkerchief or washcloth, or a foam ball, as long as it is soft (not a tennis ball).

Locate the upper insertion point of the rectus femoris: trace the iliac crest with your hand, and just in front of it, locate the anterior superior iliac spine of the pelvis. The tendon of the rectus femoris muscle is located 5 cm lower.

Situate the upper region of the rectus femoris muscle: lie on your stomach. Place the lift in the spot you just found.

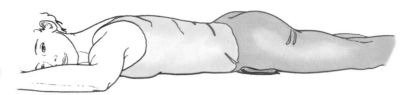

Feel how this area often forms a small hollow, and try to push on the cushion with this hollowed area. In order to push, your pelvis goes into extension and your gluteus maximus contracts. Relax and repeat several times.

Put the muscle in tension: same position. Bend one knee and take the foot in your hand.

Then feel how the hollow has formed again. Try the two stages of the preceding exercise again.

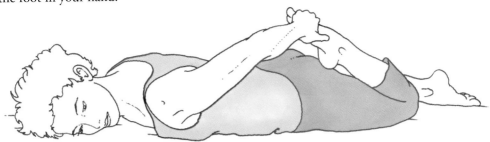

Replace the knee: the knee tends to drift outwards. If possible, place it next to your other knee.

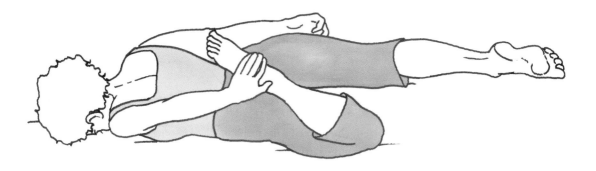

If the knee and in particular the patella (kneecap) are sensitive, the exercise will be more comfortable if you hold the foot with the help of a strap, to limit flexion in the knee.

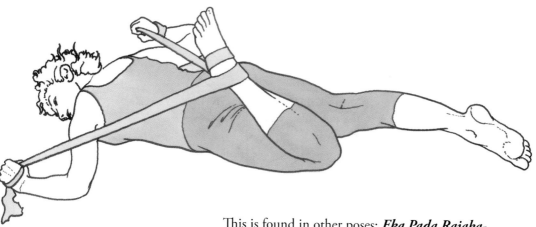

This is found in other poses: *Eka Pada Rajaka-potasana* (**One-Legged King Pigeon Pose**), *Setu Bandha Sarvangasana* (**Bridge Pose**), and *Dhanurasana* (**Bow Pose**), which simultaneously place the hip in extension and the knee in flexion.

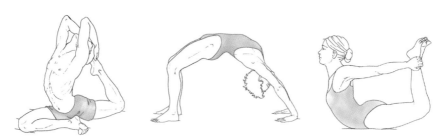

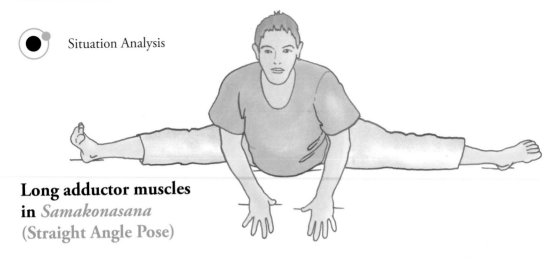

Situation Analysis

Long adductor muscles
in *Samakonasana*
(Straight Angle Pose)

When this seated pose is fully realized, the lower limbs are complete extensions of one another on each side of the pelvis. There are obviously significant differences in implementation from one person to another.

Some ligaments are stretched, which will not be discussed here. The adductor muscles are stretched, in particular the adductor magnus (AOM, p. 246).

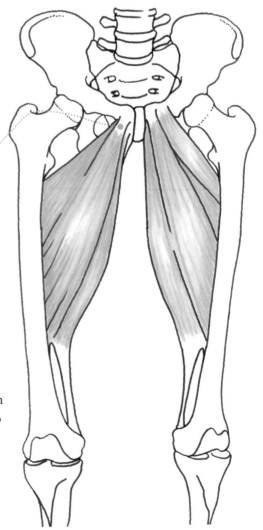

It is observed that some people, when the spread of the legs becomes intense for them, place their pelvis either in flexion or in extension. The arrangement of the adductor magnus is one of the reasons for this.

On top, this muscle attaches to the pelvis along an arm of a bone that extends from the pubis to the ischium: the ischio-pubic ramus. It is necessary here to take a good look at the orientation of this bone. From the pubis to the ischium, it descends at an angle backwards and away. The two right and left arms are symmetrical.

The adductor magnus contains:

• anterior fibers that attach quite close to the *pubis*: these fibers, when stretched by doing the splits, will pull the pelvis into flexion. The person will then settle forwards, which will lead them to lean on the hands placed in front of them;

• posterior fibers, which attach quite close to the *ischium*: these fibers, when stretched by doing the splits, will pull the pelvis into extension.

> **Locate the adductor magnus on the pelvis:** you can easily find the ischium, on which one settles when seated, and the pubis in front of the pelvis. Between these two, you can follow the ischio-pubic ramus.

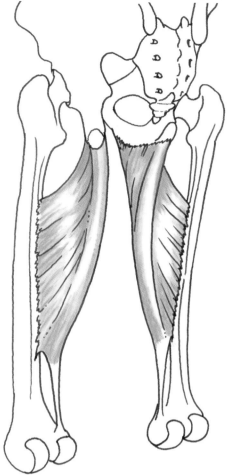

The person often drifts backwards, which leads them to instinctively lean on their hands, which are placed behind them (or, if they want to place their hands in front, it causes them to bend the trunk).

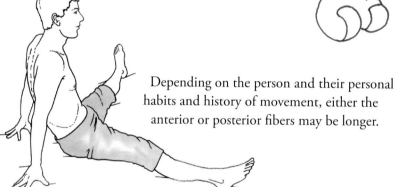

Depending on the person and their personal habits and history of movement, either the anterior or posterior fibers may be longer.

This explains the tendency to place oneself either in flexion or extension when doing the splits, without regard to the angle of opening that is achieved.

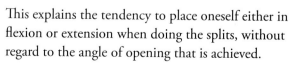
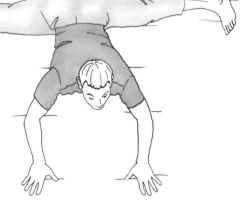

● ● ●   Stretching Exercise   •

Risk-free stretches for the adductor muscles

Caution: muscle tearing can easily occur in these muscles. They should be stretched gradually. We will play more with pelvic movements and hip rotations than with the splits themselves.

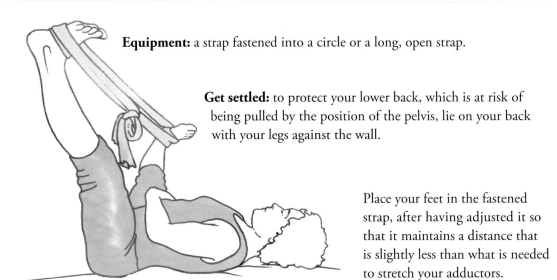

Equipment: a strap fastened into a circle or a long, open strap.

Get settled: to protect your lower back, which is at risk of being pulled by the position of the pelvis, lie on your back with your legs against the wall.

Place your feet in the fastened strap, after having adjusted it so that it maintains a distance that is slightly less than what is needed to stretch your adductors.

You can also encircle the feet with an open strap that you hold in your hands, which will allow you to adjust the distance.

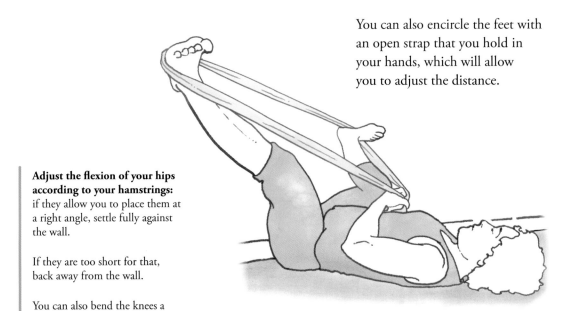

Adjust the flexion of your hips according to your hamstrings: if they allow you to place them at a right angle, settle fully against the wall.

If they are too short for that, back away from the wall.

You can also bend the knees a little, the main criterion being that you must be able to easily keep your pelvis on the ground.

Rock sideways: bring your weight onto the right buttock while easing the pressure on the left. Feel how your adductor magnus stretches on the left side.

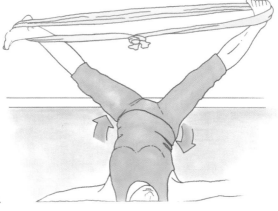

Then alternate with the other side.

Rotate the pelvis: return to a neutral position. Now rotate the pelvis horizontally on the ground, bringing the right iliac crest towards the right shoulder. Feel how your adductors stretch on the left side.

Alternate with the other side.

Flexion/extension of the pelvis (this movement will lengthen your adductors on both sides at the same time): return to a neutral position. Roll your pelvis towards the coccyx.

Then, slowly, roll it upwards towards the top of your waist: feel the stretch in the different parts of your adductors depending on the position of the pelvis.

Rotate the hips: orient your feet so that they point outwards, and then inwards. Alternate these movements several times, placing your adductor magnus in tension in different ways.

All of these movements can be repeated and alternated several times.

Other poses that stretch the adductors: *Prasarita Padottanasana* (Wide-Legged Standing Forward Bend), *Supta Baddha Konasana* (Supine Bound Angle Pose).

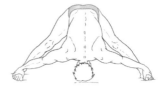
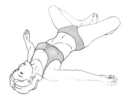

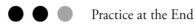 Practice at the End

A long gluteus minimus muscle
in *Padmasana* (Lotus Pose)

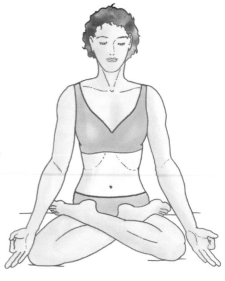

In this pose, not only do the legs cross, but each ankle comes to rest on the opposite thigh.

Each hip carries out a triple movement (illustrated here with the left hip enlarged and transparent).

At the same time, they flex significantly (a little more than 90 degrees), but not to their maximum point.

We saw on p. 114 that this requires flexibility in the gluteus maximus muscles. The hips also spread, but just slightly (the knees are barely spread in ***Padmasana***).

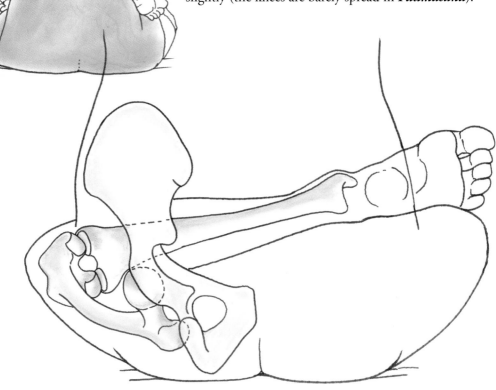

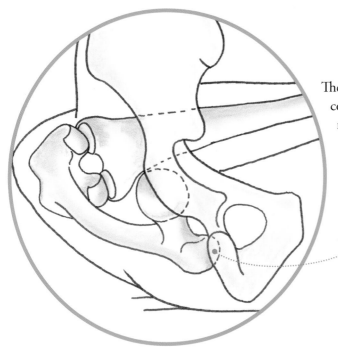

The most important movement component is that of external rotation, which is brought to its maximum point (at least 110 degrees).

The greater trochanter will sometimes even touch the ischium.

This rotation can be limited by certain ligaments, which will not be discussed here.

It can also be limited by muscles, in particular by the internal rotators of the hip, notably the gluteus minimus.

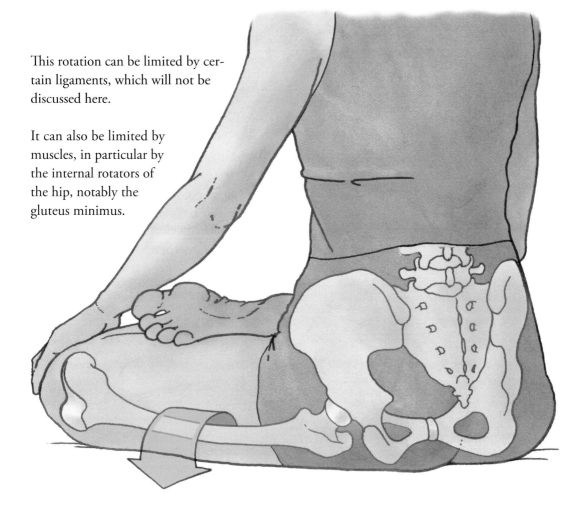

○ ○ ○   *Continued...*

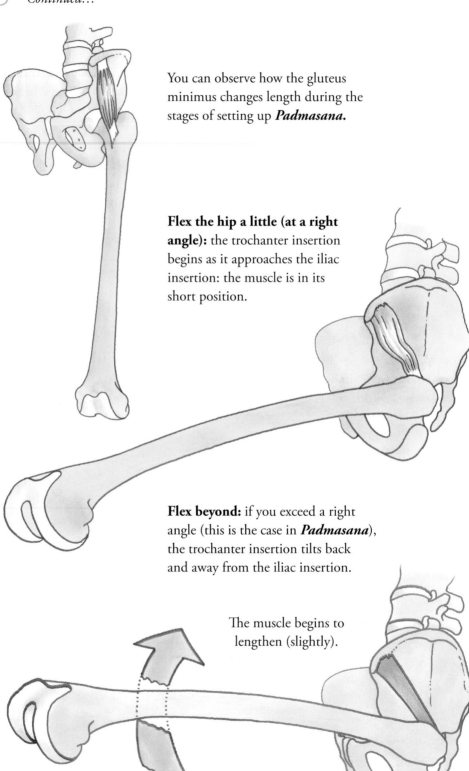

You can observe how the gluteus minimus changes length during the stages of setting up *Padmasana.*

Flex the hip a little (at a right angle): the trochanter insertion begins as it approaches the iliac insertion: the muscle is in its short position.

Flex beyond: if you exceed a right angle (this is the case in *Padmasana*), the trochanter insertion tilts back and away from the iliac insertion.

The muscle begins to lengthen (slightly).

Spread the knees a little (abduction): in this movement, the trochanter pivots towards the middle of the pelvis, stretching the gluteus minimus a little bit more.

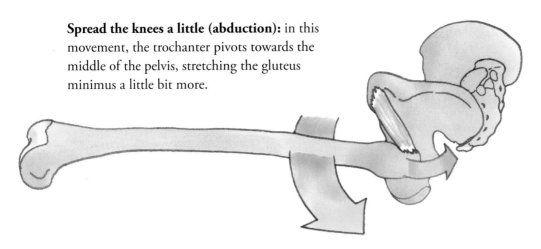

From flexion/abduction, rotate the femur considerably outwards: the trochanter pivots downwards and resides on the side of the ischium, in front of it.

It is this last movement, which is very broad, that places the gluteus minimus in maximum tension. For people who have difficulty assuming *Padmasana*, we can see that it is important to stretch the gluteus minimus, keeping in mind that it is not the sole obstacle.

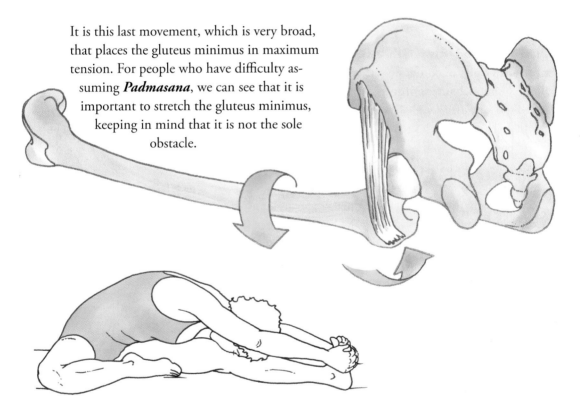

Why is **Half-Lotus** easier to practice than **Full Lotus**? If the pose is just taken on one side, the pelvis can move a little laterally and by rotating, to move the iliac insertion closer to the trochanter insertion.

This limits the stretch in the gluteus minimus, and can be a preliminary stage in achieving the pose. Be careful, however, that the pelvic movement does not become too significant, as that could cause the base of the vertebral column to become asymmetrical.

● ● ●   Stretching Exercise   · · · · · · · · · · ·   · · · · · · · ·

Stretching the gluteus minimus muscle

Equipment: a large cushion

Locate the top of the pelvis: in a standing position, find your iliac crest and its two ends (the anterior superior iliac spine and the posterior superior iliac spine).

Locate the greater trochanter: it protrudes on the side of the hip, roughly 10 centimeters below the iliac crest (if you lie on one side, the protrusion of the trochanter presses on the ground).

Place your hand between the two previous points of contact: you are in the supratrochanteric area, also called the *external iliac fossa*, where the three gluteal muscles reside.

Palpate the greater trochanter: shift your weight to one leg in order to palpate the other leg.

Feel around the greater trochanter with two fingers, recognizing its lateral aspect (insertion of the gluteus medius), its posterior aspect (insertion of the gluteus maximus), and finally the anterior aspect (insertion of the gluteus minimus).

> It is not uncommon for the tendons of these three muscles to experience pain (tendonitis) since they are constantly working when standing and walking. This may be the pain that people feel when practicing **Padmasana.** It is sometimes a sign of overworked muscles that require massaging prior to stretching.

Massage around the trochanter: to do this, lie on the side opposite the one you want to massage, placing a large cushion between your legs (or pressing the upper leg on a stool) in order to relax the muscle mass in its short position. With the heel of your hand, press across the whole area, rubbing the muscles slowly and deeply while moving forwards and backwards.

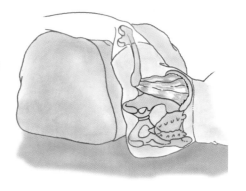

Massage and mobilize: lie on your back. Rotate your foot so that it is pointing inwards or outwards. The movement is produced in your hips, alternating between your external and internal rotators.

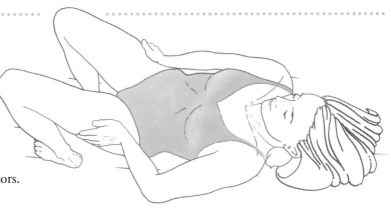

Next, return the heel of your hand to the spot between the iliac crest and the trochanter, and massage during the movement.

Do the same with the hip flexed, feet flat, and the knee moving in and out.

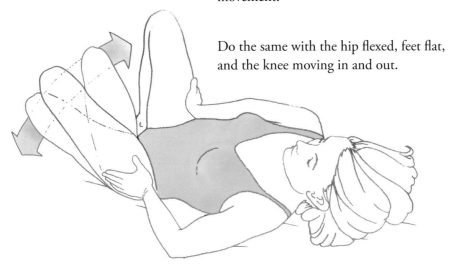

Stretching proper: *(described for the right gluteus medius)*: on your back, move your left leg 15 centimeters outwards, without changing your bearing on the pelvis (keep both buttocks on the ground). Then place your right foot where your left foot was.

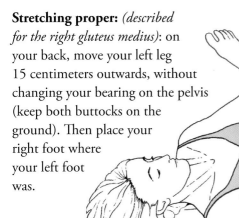

Finally, bring your left leg towards you and cross your right leg over your left. Feel how this movement (an abduction) stretches your right gluteus minimus. You can increase the stretch by raising your right arm up to the side of your head.

Practice at the End

A long pectoralis minor muscle in
Hasta Uttanasana (Raised Arms Pose)

In this pose that is a part of **Sun Salutation**, the arms are raised to the vertical, or even beyond it. This requires a certain range of motion in the shoulder joints.

Therefore, all the joints in the shoulder region participate:

The scapulae move considerably apart, gliding up on the thorax, its tip pointing forward (upward rotation, AOM, p. 115).

The clavicle is as high and as forward as possible from its joint with the sternum (the sternoclavicular joint).

The joint that connects the scapula and the clavicle (the acromioclavicular joint) is allowed to do the most to bring adaptation between the two bones.

All this makes it possible to orient the glenoid cavity of the scapula forward and upward, preparing the arm mobility from the shoulder: the humerus rises to 180 degrees, and sometimes even more.

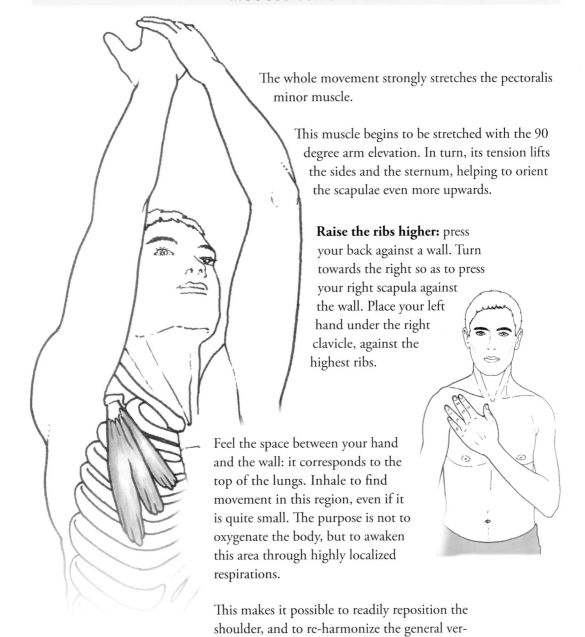

The whole movement strongly stretches the pectoralis minor muscle.

This muscle begins to be stretched with the 90 degree arm elevation. In turn, its tension lifts the sides and the sternum, helping to orient the scapulae even more upwards.

Raise the ribs higher: press your back against a wall. Turn towards the right so as to press your right scapula against the wall. Place your left hand under the right clavicle, against the highest ribs.

Feel the space between your hand and the wall: it corresponds to the top of the lungs. Inhale to find movement in this region, even if it is quite small. The purpose is not to oxygenate the body, but to awaken this area through highly localized respirations.

This makes it possible to readily reposition the shoulder, and to re-harmonize the general vertical alignment of the body.

You will find this in part in other poses: *Anjaneyasana* (**Crescent Lunge on the Knee**), *Setu Bandha Sarvangasana* (**Bridge Pose**), *Natarajasana* (**Lord of the Dance Pose**).

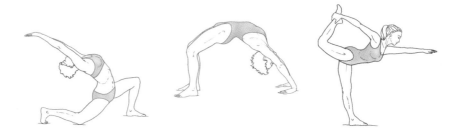

● ● ●   Stretching Exercise   ·····································

Stretching the pectoralis minor muscle

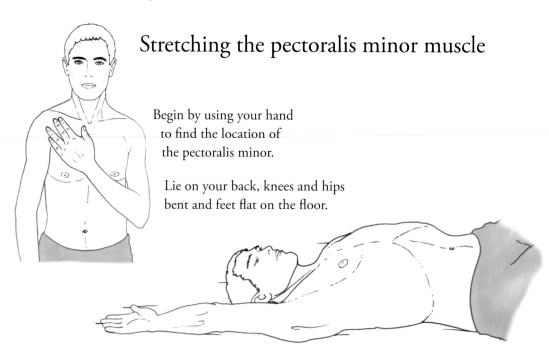

Begin by using your hand
to find the location of
the pectoralis minor.

Lie on your back, knees and hips
bent and feet flat on the floor.

Place your right arm alongside your right ear,
sliding it along the ground until the scapula
rises towards the head.

This already stretches the pectoralis minor.
To stretch it more completely, bring your
left hand to the muscle as shown above.

Unusual detail: you may raise
the shoulder along with the
arm, to elevate the coracoid
(please note that this action
only applies to this exercise).

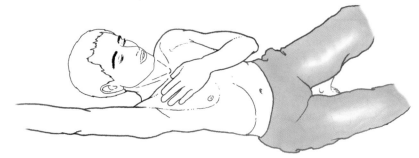

While keeping the right arm
up, exhale and send the ribs
down to this area.

Repeat on the left side.

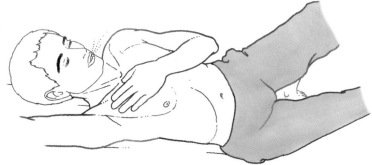

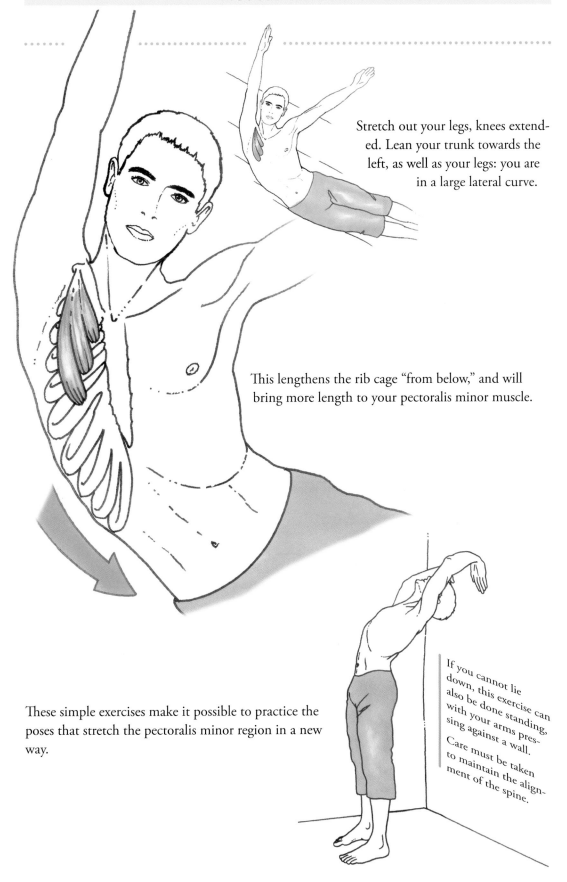

Stretch out your legs, knees extended. Lean your trunk towards the left, as well as your legs: you are in a large lateral curve.

This lengthens the rib cage "from below," and will bring more length to your pectoralis minor muscle.

These simple exercises make it possible to practice the poses that stretch the pectoralis minor region in a new way.

If you cannot lie down, this exercise can also be done standing, with your arms pressing against a wall. Care must be taken to maintain the alignment of the spine.

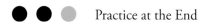

● ● ○   Practice at the End

A long and strong pectoralis major muscle in *Dhanurasana* (Bow Pose)

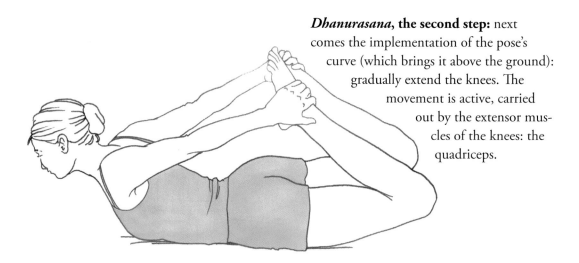

Bow is a "bound" pose: the hands hold the ankles. As always in such cases, the range required in the joints can be distributed and shifted from one to the other, here in particular towards *the shoulder*.

We will observe forward and backward shoulder movements (here we will use "shoulder" to mean the collection of joints that facilitate arm movements, without going into detail).

Forwards and backwards, they perform two kinds of movement: flexion, towards the front, which has a very broad range (up to 180 degrees), and extension, towards the back, which is much more limited, generally reaching 45 degrees.

Dhanurasana, **the first step:** you start by lying on the stomach. Bend the knees by bringing the feet towards the buttocks. The arms stretch back, elbows extended, to grasp each ankle with the hands. Many parts of the body are on the ground. The joints are in moderate range, except the knees, which are quite bent.

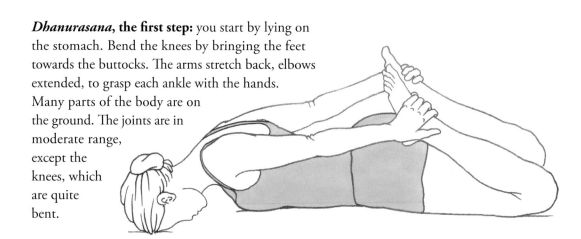

Dhanurasana, **the second step:** next comes the implementation of the pose's curve (which brings it above the ground): gradually extend the knees. The movement is active, carried out by the extensor muscles of the knees: the quadriceps.

Three types of compensation: to practice this pose we unfold the knees, and so range of flexion is lost. But since the pose is "bound," what is lost in the knees must be made up for elsewhere, more precisely in three possible areas:

- either in the hips, where greater extension is required,

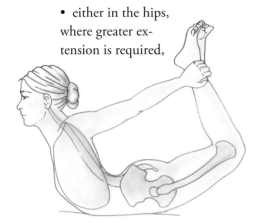

- or in the lumbar spine, where greater arching is required,

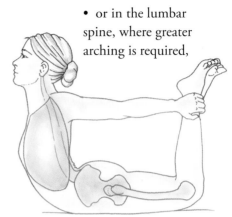

- or in the shoulder, where we ask for more backward movement:

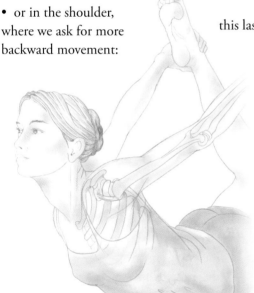

this last alternative is detailed here.

The extension of the shoulder increases sharply. It will reach — and sometimes exceed — 45 degrees. This strongly stretches the ligaments as well as the anterior muscles of the shoulder.

If the extension is significant, it will be hampered by the muscles situated in front of the joint, in particular the pectoralis major (AOM, p. 124). This muscle, a large layer spreading from the front of the thorax to the humerus, is a powerful cinch for the shoulder.

To protect the joint, it is both completely stretched and contracted. This pose thus requires the pectoralis major to be both strong (for restraint) and supple (to allow range in the arm).

Why is the asymmetrical *Bow Pose* (One-Legged Upward Bow) easier on the shoulder? Because the pelvis and the thorax perform a twist that reduces the range needed in the front of the shoulder and in the hip.

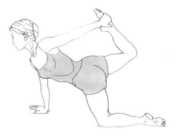

Stretching the pectoralis major

Position yourself: lie on your back with the hips, knees and heels bent, feet flat on the ground. Spread your arms wide to each side.

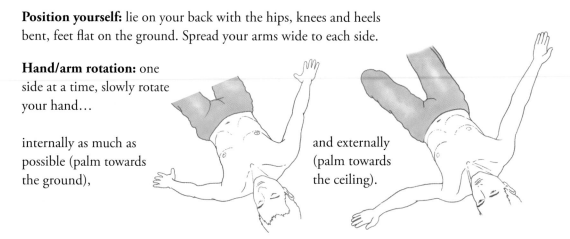

Hand/arm rotation: one side at a time, slowly rotate your hand…

internally as much as possible (palm towards the ground),

and externally (palm towards the ceiling).

Make it so this movement not only occurs in the hand and the forearm, but in the whole arm starting from the shoulder.

Raise the arm: slide one arm up to the level of your ear or forehead. Feel how the pectoralis major is gradually placed in tension. You can palpate it at its upper insertion.

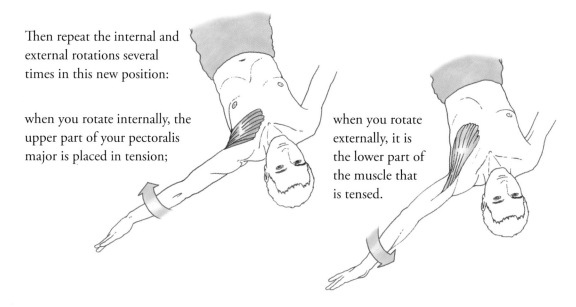

Then repeat the internal and external rotations several times in this new position:

when you rotate internally, the upper part of your pectoralis major is placed in tension;

when you rotate externally, it is the lower part of the muscle that is tensed.

Head/neck and the front of the thorax: slowly turn the head to one side. Feel how the top of your thorax tends to rotate to the same side and to press down more.

On the opposite side, the shoulder has a (slight) tendency to decrease its pressure on the ground, and this tenses the pectoralis major on this side. Be sure to keep your arm in contact with the ground as much as possible.

Twisted legs (*described for the right pectoralis major*): keep your left foot on the ground. Place your right leg on your left knee.

Take your right knee, bent as pictured, towards the ground on the left side.

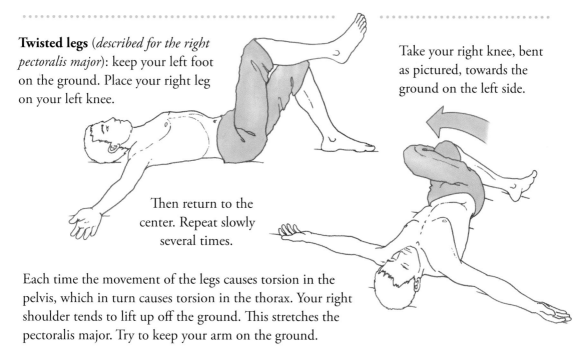

Then return to the center. Repeat slowly several times.

Each time the movement of the legs causes torsion in the pelvis, which in turn causes torsion in the thorax. Your right shoulder tends to lift up off the ground. This stretches the pectoralis major. Try to keep your arm on the ground.

At first, do not go far with the legs, so as not to pull the shoulder very much. Gradually increase the movement, always aiming for comfort in the front of your shoulder. Here too, try orienting the arm in two ways: internally and externally.

Stretching the pectoralis major while standing (*described for the right pectoralis major*):

Place yourself perpendicular to a wall, the right shoulder towards the wall. Lift your right arm and place the palm of your hand against the wall, facing backward.

Feel how this placement places your pectoralis major in tension. You can increase this stretch by turning your thorax to the left.

You can also turn your head to the left.

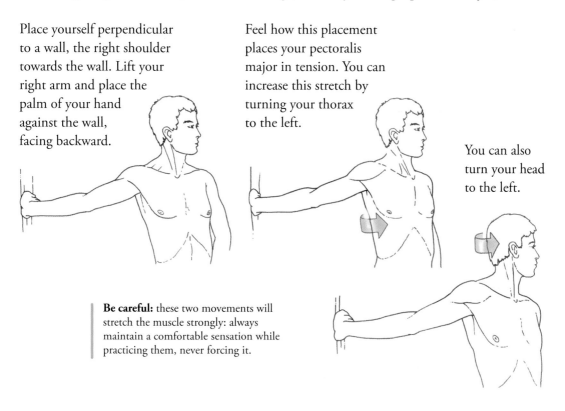

Be careful: these two movements will stretch the muscle strongly: always maintain a comfortable sensation while practicing them, never forcing it.

Practice at the End

A long triceps brachii muscle in
Gomukhasana (Cow Face Pose)

In this pose, the arms make inverse movements in the shoulders. Their ranges of motion determine the ease of movement as well as the benefit for the shoulders, especially when the hands are clasped.

Here we will observe the upper arm in the pose: it is placed vertically and the shoulder is rotated externally. The elbow is greatly flexed. The range of the two joints is maximal.

In *Gomukhasana*, the scapulae rotate upwards (AOM, p. 115). There are two reasons for this:

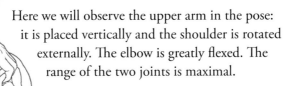

first the tension of the capsule, but also the tension of the long head of the triceps brachii.

This large muscle, consisting of three parts (called the three "heads"), attaches at the back of the arm and extends farther on the bone to the point of the elbow (AOM, p. 148). The strong elbow flexion stretches it.

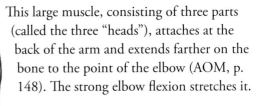

But **Gomukhasana** primarily stretches one of the muscle's heads, called the *long head*. In fact, the bending of the elbow occurs simultaneously with the elevation of the arm.

However, this long head extends up to the scapula. And when it is placed in tension, it pulls the scapula in upward rotation.

If the long head is shortened, the shoulder will lack range and the upward rotation becomes significant.

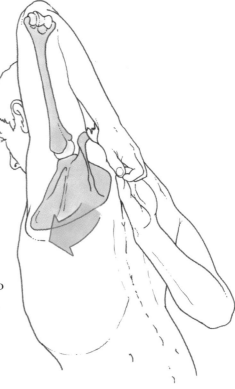

We then see, under the arm, a protruding mass: it is the scapula, which has become almost horizontal, its tip directed forward and out.

We can also see that the arm cannot go backwards and that it pushes the head forward.

○ ○ ○ *Continued…*

You can prepare for the movement of the upper arms in **Gomukhasana**
by stretching the long head of the triceps brachii.

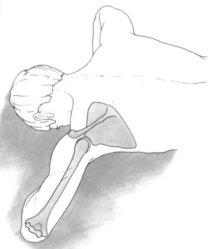

Setup: lie on your stomach, and place your arms
on either side of your head, the elbows bent and
the hands close to the ears.

Find downward rotation of the scapulae:
without moving your hands too much,
glide your elbows towards your waist:
your arms approach the trunk.

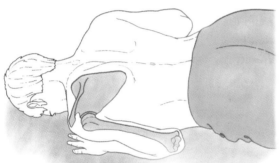

Feel how your scapulae move closer to
your spine. They perform a downward
rotation, which primarily moves their
point towards the median line of the
back.

Find upward rotation: slowly
spread the scapulae again, to feel
what they do: the point is now
outside the median line. This is
upward rotation.

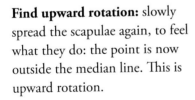

Active version: practice these two movements several times to really feel how the scapulae are
first pulled into the arm movement. Then perform them with just the scapulae, without moving
the arms: they are then performed actively by the muscles.

Repeat the active downward rotation several times, as this will be necessary in the next exercise.

Extend the arm on the floor *(described for the left arm)*: slide the right arm along the floor beyond your head, in an extension of your body.

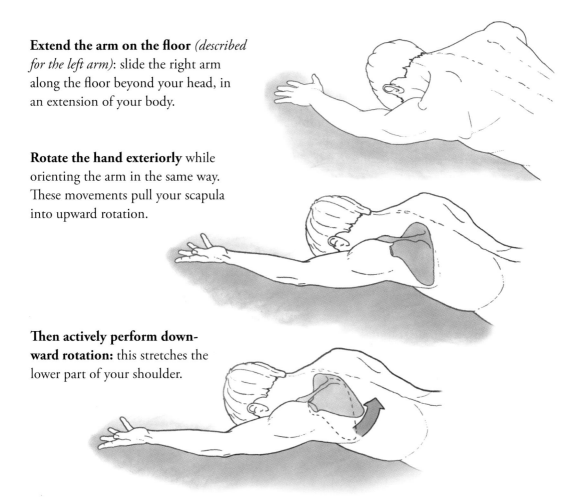

Rotate the hand exteriorly while orienting the arm in the same way. These movements pull your scapula into upward rotation.

Then actively perform down-ward rotation: this stretches the lower part of your shoulder.

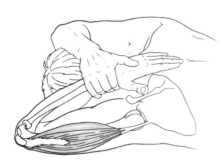

Regain elbow flexion: bend your elbow. Use the other hand to gently maintain or increase this flexion. The up-ward rotation tends to become stronger: this is due to the stretching of the long head. Then actively re-direct your scapula into downward rotation. Next, move your arm and shoulder.

You can prepare your shoulder for several sessions before putting it into practice in ***Gomukhasana***.

Other poses where we find the same stretches: *Natarajasana* **(Lord of the Dance Pose)**, *Eka Pada Rajakapotasana* **(One-Legged King Pigeon Pose)**, *Dhanurasana* **(Bow Pose)**.

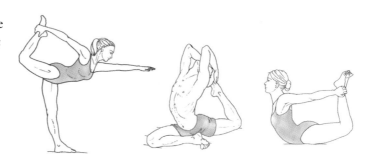

Long rhomboid muscles as a result of *Garudasana* (Eagle Pose)

The elbows are crossed in certain variants of this pose, which strongly spreads the shoulders from behind. This allows you to find range between the scapulae, to breathe, and to free up the neck and upper back.

First we will observe the area.

The movements of the scapula: this bone is not attached by a joint in back, but is connected to the spine and the rib cage by six muscles with complementary actions which mobilize or stabilize it, two roles determined by the arms and the hand.

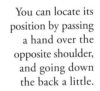

The rhomboids, from the scapulae to the spine: between them, the rhomboids (AOM, p. 82) go from the medial border of the scapula to the cervical and thoracic vertebrae.

It approaches the spine while moving upwards. Like an active cinch, it holds the scapula, in back, and prevents it from moving away from the spine.

You can locate its position by passing a hand over the opposite shoulder, and going down the back a little.

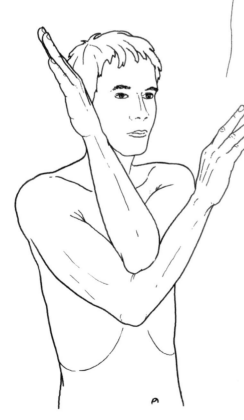

We can observe the **Garudasana** arms: they are crossed in front of the chest, one of the arms placed under the other with the elbow bent. This stretches the scapulae firmly apart (abduction).

The positioning of the arms could finish with this first movement, and the arms would then be in internal rotation at the shoulder.

But a second movement is added to the pose:

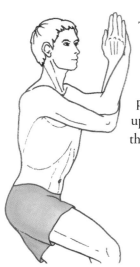

The hands come back towards one another, which turns the arms in external rotation, and the position is then "locked up" with the clasping of the hands.

This additional detail further spreads the scapulae. The rhomboids are thus strongly stretched, especially their upper part.

This stretching is relevant in two situations, which can be exercises that follow the pose.

1) Posterior breathing:

• Round the dorsal region, including the upper dorsal region between the scapulae.

• Inhale as if you are trying to send the air to this posterior area (this is a visual aid, but it most often works when finding the location of a breathing movement).

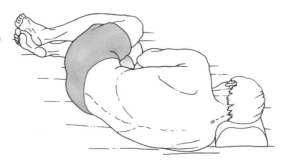

• Repeat during several inhalations, without forcing, but aiming instead for ease and comfort in this area.

2) Ease the neck. After practicing *Garudasana*, explore the mobility of the base of your neck:

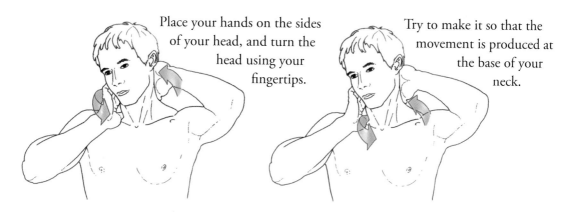

Place your hands on the sides of your head, and turn the head using your fingertips.

Try to make it so that the movement is produced at the base of your neck.

Situation Analysis

A stretched diaphragm in
Sarvangasana (Shoulderstand)

In this pose, you roll up the legs
and then the trunk until you…

…are vertically erect and
balancing on the shoulders.

The pelvis and the ribcage are in an inverted
position. Of all the things that this causes
to happen in the body, here we will
look at two in particular:

• for one thing, the internal
organs of the abdomen tend
to slide towards the head,

• and at the same time, the
lower part of the ribcage becomes like a receptacle with
just the right shape to collect
them in.

The weight of the visceral mass is, in fact,
received by the sheet of muscle called the
diaphragm (AOM, p. 90).

Its domed shape, in an inverted position, acts
like a large pliant bowl in which the internal
organs come to support themselves in a
flexible way.

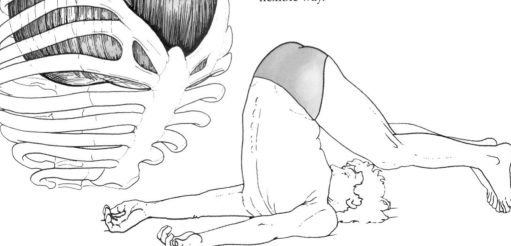

The diaphragm reacts to this pressure by contracting a little. But at the same time, the weight of the internal organs pushes it (moderately) towards the head: this stretches the muscle fibers.

The stretching of the diaphragm is useful for ease of breathing, since the muscle thus contains greater range between its contracted position (inhaling) and uncontracted position (exhaling).

This is found in most inverted poses.

Note: it is a mistake to believe that the steeper the slope, the greater the effect. This is because the gliding of the internal organs is balanced by the contraction of the muscles that hold the trunk tightly all the way around it.

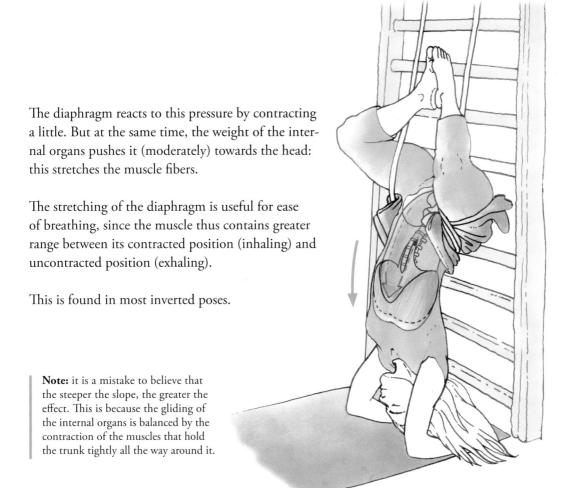

Conversely, the effect is stronger if the pose is modified with a support under the pelvis (a block placed under the pelvis, or cushions forming a support like a toboggan). Why?

Because then, in the trunk, it is not necessary to "hold" the pose with contractions of the local muscles (the abdominal muscles, among others), and the sliding of the internal organs is not hindered by this tonicity.

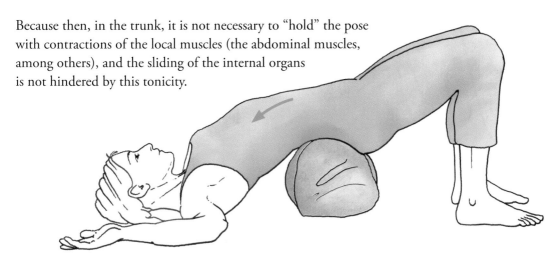

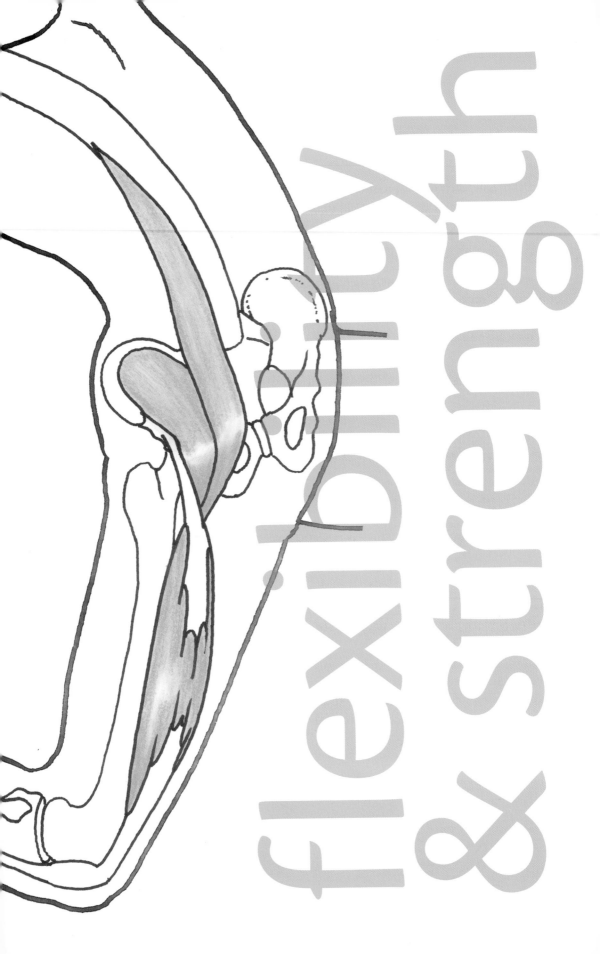

flexibility & strength

5

Flexibility & Strength in Certain Poses

Chapter 2 dealt with strength, and Chapter 4 with muscular flexibility. This chapter considers the case of poses that *necessitate, as a prerequisite, the length in certain muscles, so that the strength of other muscles can be effectively implemented.*

If the muscles that require length do in fact possess it, then the pose can be performed. The action of the "pose-building muscles" can be accomplished.

But, if the muscles that require length are (as of yet) too short, there are two possible ways to manage this:

• either we try *to assume the correct form of the pose anyway.* We then implement muscular actions to "overcome the stiffness" of muscles that are too short. The yoga practice is thus monopolized by this fight against these obstacles (a little like trying to move in a garment that is too short).

• or we can *adapt the pose to the muscular stiffness, without changing the stiffness.* But this demands too much range of motion from the neighboring joints. The pose no longer has the same form. This practice may carry risks.

THE FOLLOWING PAGES will present five poses for which flexibility is considered indispensable to the active construction of the pose.

Note   When it comes to muscular flexibility, people are not completely equal (the same goes for ligamental flexibility). Faced with certain poses, some beginners will not have any major problems, while others will find it impossible to practice the pose. In the osteoarticular chain involved in a movement, there is sometimes great risk of demanding too much range of motion from a joint to compensate for a muscle's lack of flexibility.

5 Themed Explanation Sheets: Poses Discussed

Situation Analysis

Flexibility in the hamstrings for exerting the strength of the psoas and quadriceps in *Navasana* (Boat Pose) with straight knees

This pose (see p. 56) demands a great deal of abdominal muscle strength, as well as back muscle strength (to stabilize the pelvis and to keep the trunk erect), psoas strength (to flex the thighs), and quadricep strength (to extend the knees).

If you want to practice this pose with your knees straight, your hamstring muscles will be tensed (by the flexion of the hip combined with the extension of the knee).

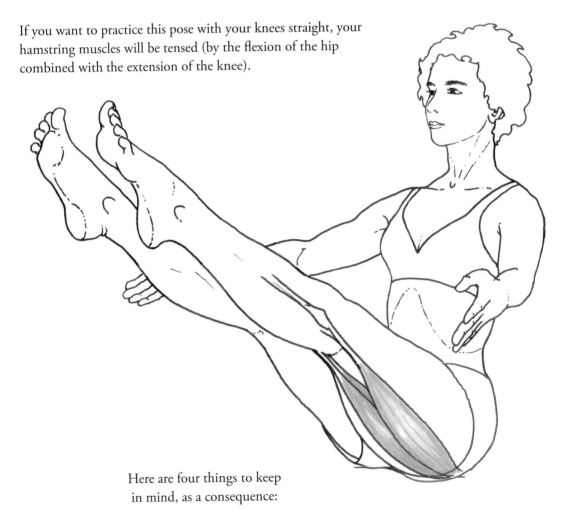

Here are four things to keep in mind, as a consequence:

1. It is difficult to keep the knees straight: the hamstring muscles, when placed in tension, pull the tibia and the fibula into flexion.

Your quadriceps thus work simultaneously to lift the tibia and to overcome the tension in the backs of the thighs.

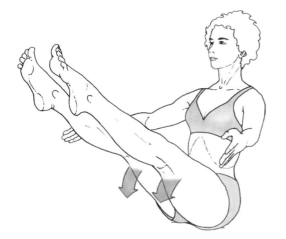

2. You need a lot more strength to flex the thighs: your hamstring muscles pull the thighs towards the ground. Your psoas and iliacus muscles work both to lift the thighs together with the entire leg, as well as to overcome the tension in the backs of the thighs.

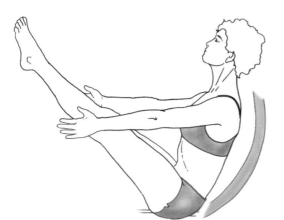

3. Your pelvis tends to go into extension: it is also pulled by the hamstrings. Therefore, either the back muscles or the hip flexors must work to balance the pelvis in a neutral position on the ischia. This increases the intensity of the abdominal muscles' work.

4. Your head drifts forward: extension of the pelvis impacts the whole trunk, which then has a tendency to flex.

To compensate, your head tends to move forward.

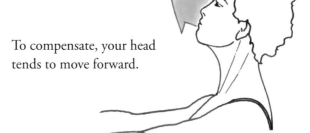

If the hamstring muscles lack sufficient length, maintaining this pose with straightened knees requires disproportionate muscle strength. It is therefore necessary to stretch the hamstring muscles before making any attempt to practice *Navasana* with straight knees.

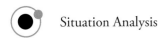

Situation Analysis

Flexiblity in the pectoral muscles for exerting the strength of the deltoid muscles in *Salabhasana* (Locust Pose) with arms extended in front

This pose (see p. 60 for the version with arms alongside the body) requires significant strength from the trunk extensor muscles (to straighten the back) and the neck (to lift the head).

If you want to practice this pose with your arms raised in front of your head, this will place the pectoralis major muscles in tension (through retropulsion of the humerus).

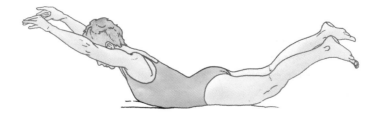

Consider two things that will increase as a result:

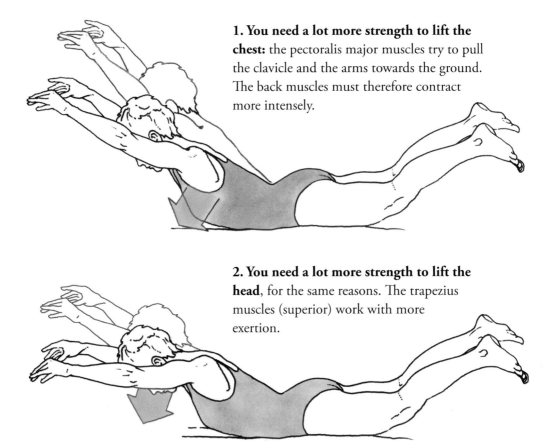

1. You need a lot more strength to lift the chest: the pectoralis major muscles try to pull the clavicle and the arms towards the ground. The back muscles must therefore contract more intensely.

2. You need a lot more strength to lift the head, for the same reasons. The trapezius muscles (superior) work with more exertion.

For the actual elevation of the arms: your deltoid muscles (posterior) and trapezius muscles are contracted. This is especially true if, in front, the pectoralis major and minor are short. If this is the case, they must work simultaneously to lift the arms and to overcome the tension in the pectoral muscles.

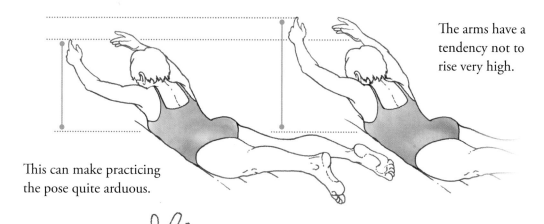

The arms have a tendency not to rise very high.

This can make practicing the pose quite arduous.

If the pectoral muscles do not have sufficient length (which you can test by simply raising the arm),

this pose with extended arms requires disproportionate strength in the arm muscles, which can make it quite arduous to practice.

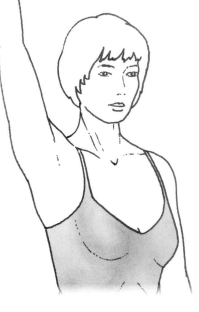

It would therefore be preferable to stretch the pectoral muscles (sometimes with assistance, see pp. 140 and 144) before making any attempt to practice **Salabhasana** with extended arms.

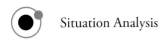

Situation Analysis

Flexibility in the shoulders, the trunk, and the hips in *Natarajasana* (Lord of the Dance)

In this pose, grasp your foot from behind with your hand, creating a kind of circle between the bended arm, the extended trunk, and the leg bent at the knee. This "circle" is balanced on one foot. The chest, together with the whole trunk, leans more or less forward.

Natarajasana **(Lord of the Dance)** assumes several flexibility prerequisites:

The front of the hip must allow a significant extension of the joint.

This is in connection with the anterior ligaments, which must possess sufficient length. It is also due to the rectus femoris, which is stretched when the hip is extended while the knee is simultaneously in flexion (see stretches for this muscle on p. 126). But it also has to do with the psoas, which must allow the extension of the hip to extend into the lumbar region (for the psoas muscle, see p. 122).

If these three elements lack length, the extension risks dominating the lower lumbar region, at the point of transition between the pelvis and the lumbar vertebrae.

The front of the shoulder must be able to send the arm far back.

At the muscular level, this changes according to the variant of the pose:

• if the arm passes back over the shoulder to grasp the foot, extension is primarily necessary in the pectoralis minor (see stretches for this muscle, p. 140);

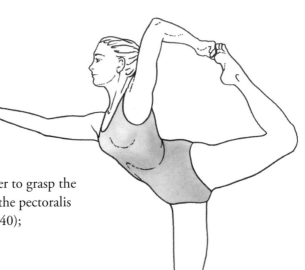

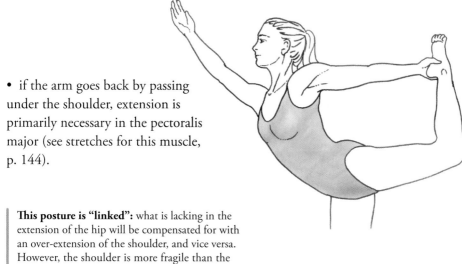

• if the arm goes back by passing under the shoulder, extension is primarily necessary in the pectoralis major (see stretches for this muscle, p. 144).

> **This posture is "linked":** what is lacking in the extension of the hip will be compensated for with an over-extension of the shoulder, and vice versa. However, the shoulder is more fragile than the hip when stretched too intensely.

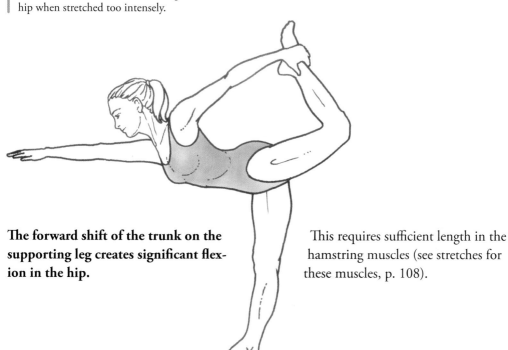

The forward shift of the trunk on the supporting leg creates significant flexion in the hip.

This requires sufficient length in the hamstring muscles (see stretches for these muscles, p. 108).

If the extensions in the front of the lifted hip, the shoulder, and the back of the supporting hip are not sufficient, the circle cannot be completed and it will be impossible to "perch" on the supporting leg.

Practicing the pose would then require disproportionate strength from the posterior muscles, which could make it quite arduous. It would therefore be preferable to stretch the prerequisite muscles before making any attempt to practice *Natarajasana*.

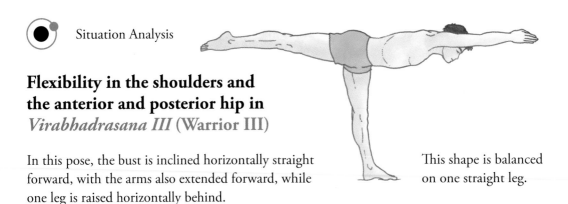

○ Situation Analysis

Flexibility in the shoulders and the anterior and posterior hip in *Virabhadrasana III* (Warrior III)

In this pose, the bust is inclined horizontally straight forward, with the arms also extended forward, while one leg is raised horizontally behind.

This shape is balanced on one straight leg.

This requires intense contractions as well as several prerequisite flexibilities.

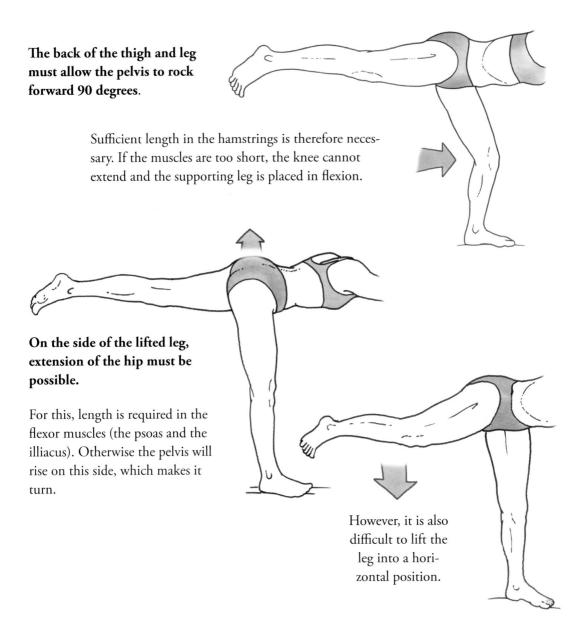

The back of the thigh and leg must allow the pelvis to rock forward 90 degrees.

Sufficient length in the hamstrings is therefore necessary. If the muscles are too short, the knee cannot extend and the supporting leg is placed in flexion.

On the side of the lifted leg, extension of the hip must be possible.

For this, length is required in the flexor muscles (the psoas and the illiacus). Otherwise the pelvis will rise on this side, which makes it turn.

However, it is also difficult to lift the leg into a horizontal position.

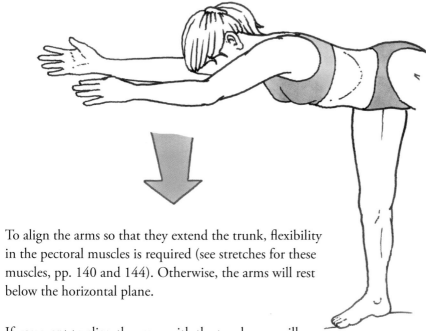

To align the arms so that they extend the trunk, flexibility in the pectoral muscles is required (see stretches for these muscles, pp. 140 and 144). Otherwise, the arms will rest below the horizontal plane.

If you want to align the arms with the trunk, you will need significant strength in the posterior deltoid muscles.

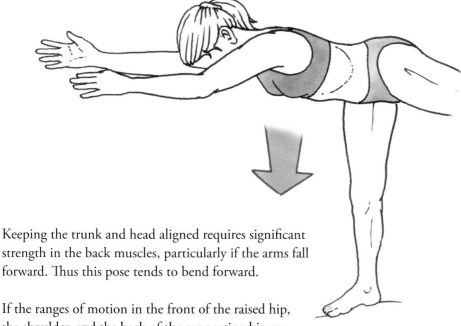

Keeping the trunk and head aligned requires significant strength in the back muscles, particularly if the arms fall forward. Thus this pose tends to bend forward.

If the ranges of motion in the front of the raised hip, the shoulder, and the back of the supporting hip are not sufficient, it is difficult or even quite arduous to bring about the horizontal alignment of the pose, as this requires disproportionate strength to fight against the areas of muscular stiffness. It is therefore important to prepare the necessary flexibility before practicing *Virabhadrasana III* (**Warrior III**).

Situation Analysis

Flexibility in the shoulders, the hips, and the thighs for exerting strength in *Chakrasana* (Wheel Pose)

This pose involves pushing the trunk away from the ground, using the strength of the limbs.

Begin in **Half-Bridge Pose**, which lifts the pelvis, then push through the hands to raise the ribcage and the head.

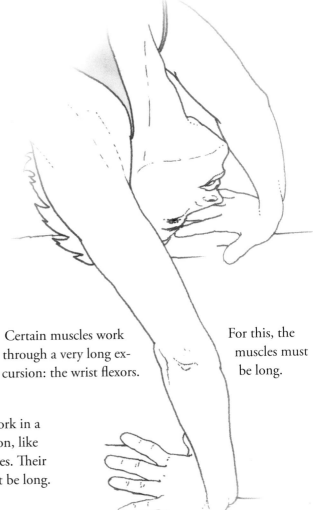

Apart from anchoring the wrists and the ankles that repel the mat, it also employs extension of the knees (quadriceps) and the elbows (triceps brachii), but above all the extension of the hips (gluteal muscles) and the retropulsion of the arms (posterior deltoids and scapula fixators: rhomboids, serratus anterior)

Certain muscles work through a very long excursion: the wrist flexors.

For this, the muscles must be long.

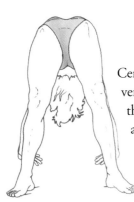

Certain muscles work in a very short excursion, like the gluteal muscles. Their antagonists must be long.

At the same time that strength is exerted, the complete execution of the pose requires that:

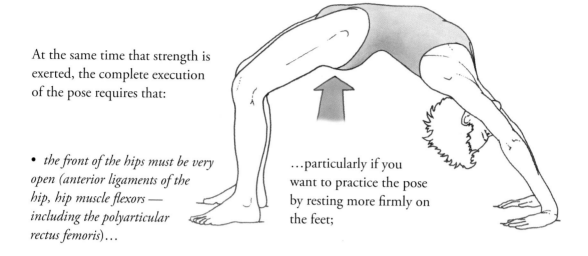

- *the front of the hips must be very open (anterior ligaments of the hip, hip muscle flexors — including the polyarticular rectus femoris)…*

…particularly if you want to practice the pose by resting more firmly on the feet;

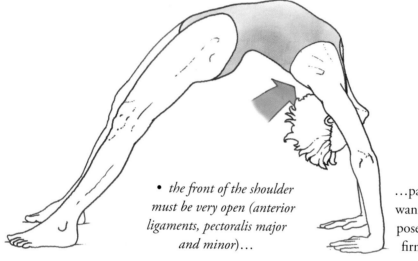

- *the front of the shoulder must be very open (anterior ligaments, pectoralis major and minor)…*

…particularly if you want to practice the pose by resting more firmly on the hands;

- *the front of the rib cage must be very open* (in terms of the dorsal spine extension) to avoid the curve being taken on exclusively by the L5 joint.

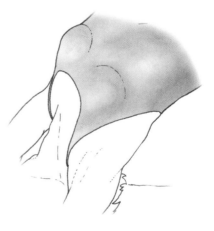

If these areas are not made flexible, muscular strength will be largely depleted in fighting against the "brakes" at the front of the body. It is therefore necessary to work on the required flexibility long in advance of practicing **Chakrasana**.

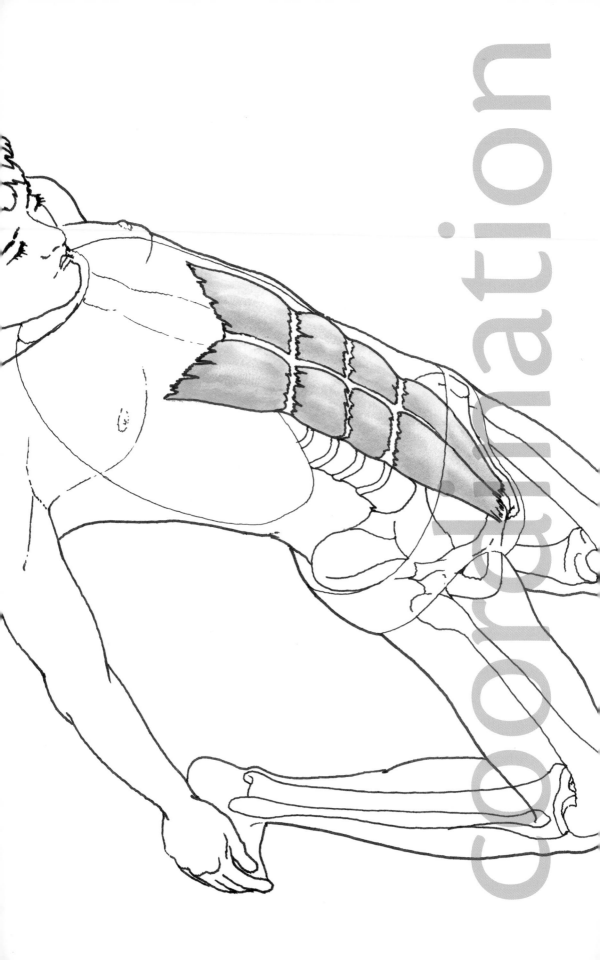

6

Muscle Coordination in the Poses

One typical feature of yoga is having to *maintain* a pose. In this moment, we can of course be attentive to our breath, our thoughts, etc. But also, the situation allows plenty of time to *adjust the placement of each part of the body*. This is a form of mini-movement.

On each joint,* the muscles play a role of active adjustment for the orientation of the bones. This leaves traces of memory, or know-how, which subsequently becomes routine.

The details of skeletal and articular placement thus become ever-more refined and complete. This is a different role from that of pure strength, which measures out the contraction necessary — neither too much nor too little — and the muscle synergy that matches this amount.

This allows for different functions according to the circumstances: protecting a joint or a nerve, orienting a bone, supporting a body part, sometimes suspending it…

---

* Inasmuch as it has the necessary range of motion.

THE FOLLOWING PAGES will present nine examples where the role of muscular contraction is essentially to "adjust" the precision of the movement.

9 Themed Explanation Sheets: 8 Poses Discussed

● ● ● Intermittent Practice

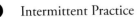

Balance the muscles forward and backward in
Tadasana (Mountain Pose)

Tadasana is like the beginning of all the standing poses. Here we will observe the moment preceding the pose, when, standing, you oscillate back and forth in order to figure out how to distribute the weight of your body on the feet. Within the space of a few degrees the pose feels quite different, either stimulating or relaxed.

Oscillate as a unit: try to oscillate solely *from your ankles*, and keep the rest of your body above the ankles as straight as possible...

without bending in the hips or knees,

or creating movements in the spine.

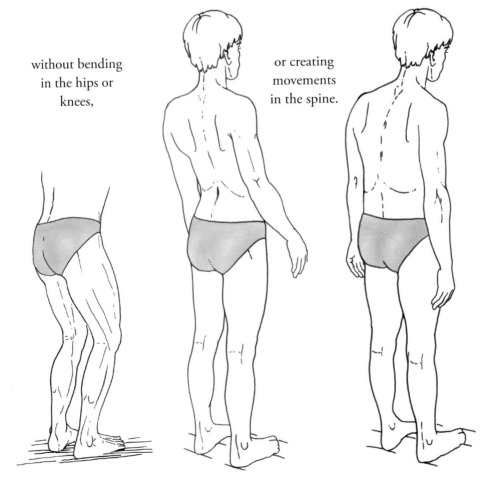

Observe this oscillation on two levels:

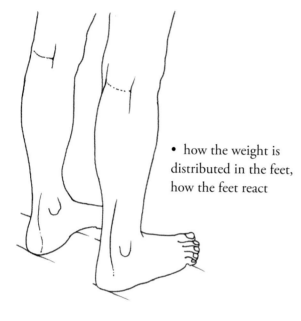

• how the weight is distributed in the feet, how the feet react

• how the body as a whole reacts by engaging the balancing muscles.

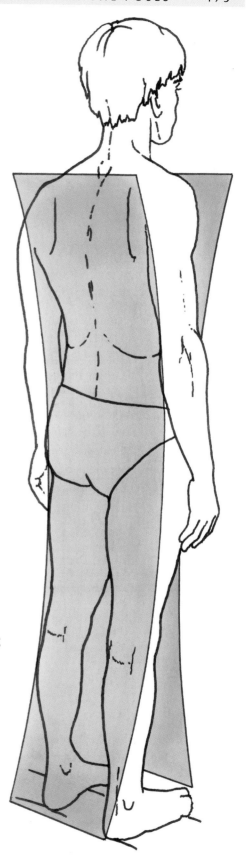

○ ○ ○   *Continued…*

First practice large oscillations. Rock quite far, to the edge of your balance. Move slowly, and stop for several seconds once the incline is at its maximum.

Anterior balance "limit:" go far forward.

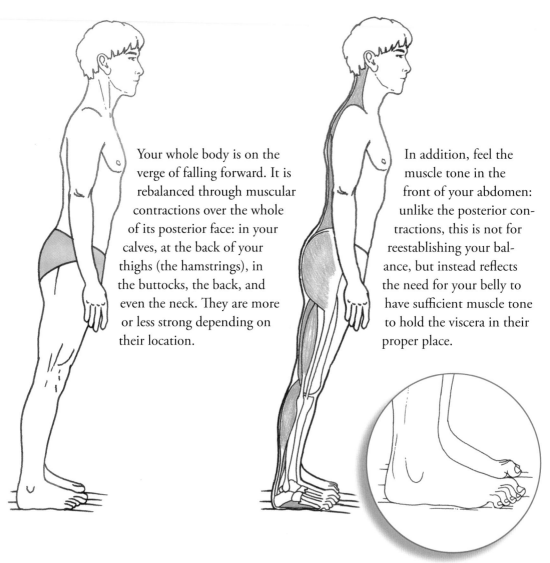

Your whole body is on the verge of falling forward. It is rebalanced through muscular contractions over the whole of its posterior face: in your calves, at the back of your thighs (the hamstrings), in the buttocks, the back, and even the neck. They are more or less strong depending on their location.

In addition, feel the muscle tone in the front of your abdomen: unlike the posterior contractions, this is not for reestablishing your balance, but instead reflects the need for your belly to have sufficient muscle tone to hold the viscera in their proper place.

In the feet, *you barely press on the heels*, mostly pressing through the front of the foot. Your toes tend to "cling" to the ground, as if clawing at it.

The bottoms of your feet are very contracted.

Come back, and do several oscillations in a faster manner in order to regain a neutral tone before the second step.

Posterior balance "limit": go as far back as possible (without "arching" at the waist). You will reach the limit more quickly: in back, there is no foot to push back on.

In the feet, feel how your weight comes to *your heels*, and even to the back of them. Your toes tend to rise strongly. It is the tops of your feet that are contracted: the tendons protrude up to the toes.

Your whole body is on the verge of falling backward. You rebalance it through *intense contractions over the whole of its anterior face:* these are the muscles that correspond to the tendons protruding from your feet, and the front of your thighs (the quadriceps).

Higher up, your abdominal muscles are maximally engaged, not only for holding in the internal organs, but in order to retain the skeletal structure of the trunk, which would otherwise bend back.

If you maintain this extreme balance, you will even feel the muscles at the front of your neck contract.

○ ○ ○   *Continued…*

The two previous oscillations are extreme. They constitute an exploration, for feeling the muscle engagement in each one. They are not suitable for staying in ***Tadasana***. Between these, experiment with two more moderate positions.

First come back, through a few oscillations, to a neutral position.

Comfortably balance to the back: place three-quarters of your weight on the heel, and one-quarter on the fore-foot (without pressing on the toes).

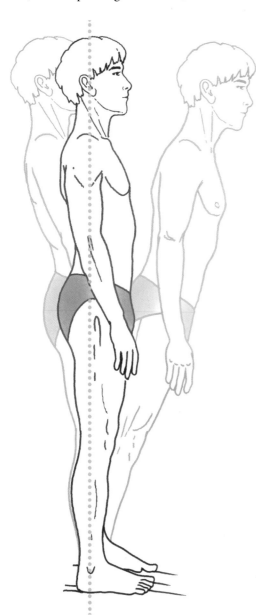

This position allows a certain muscular rest:

• the arch of the foot is not strongly loaded, since the weight is on the solid bones of the hindfoot. Result: the muscles that support this arch relax (a little).

• the tibia is placed vertically on the foot. It balances itself with tiny contractions. Above, the femur can settle vertically on the tibia.

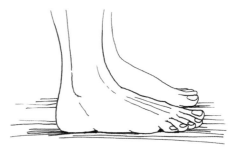

It is therefore a very "economical" posture from a muscular point of view, where you stand with minimal effort "on the bones." It is relaxing and appropriate for long-duration standing poses. The balance here is quite fine: you are not very far from falling back, which requires an adjustment of the bones of the hindfoot that must be placed precisely one over (or under) the other.

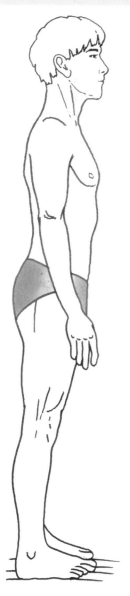

Comfortably balance to the front: bring 50% of your weight to the heels, and 50% to the forefoot.

There, muscular work is more significant since:

• you have "charged" the arch of the foot: the muscles that support it are contracted in order to maintain it;

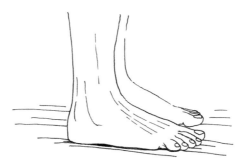

• your tibia is no longer vertical, but rather is at a bit of an angle to the foot. Your triceps surae contract to restore balance. This position is therefore more "muscular." The balance here is easier: you can go a little forward or backward and the posterior muscles simply contract more or less.

It is not a resting position but rather one of moderate muscle toning.

By changing your oscillation a few degrees in *Tadasana*, you can switch from the third to the fourth position and vice versa. The sensations are quite different. Depending on the context of the practice, you may prefer a "skeletal" balance — fine, almost relaxed — or a "muscular" balance, which is more toning.

Other poses where we find these muscular actions: all the other standing poses: *Vrikshasana* (**Tree Pose**), *Garudasana* (**Eagle Pose**), *Natarajasana* (**Lord of the Dance Pose**).

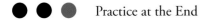 Practice at the End

Contract the multifidus muscle to distribute the movement in *Marichiasana* (Seated Spinal Twist)

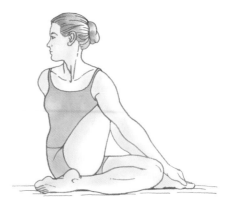

This pose has many variations. Here we will observe those which rotate the spine (torsion) by first identifying that the possibility for this movement is not present everywhere in the spine.

Torsion does not exist in the lumbar spine.

We can observe the trunk from the bottom up. The first vertebrae, in the waist region, are the lumbar vertebrae.

At the back, their shape is one of joints interlocking vertically like sections of cylinders.

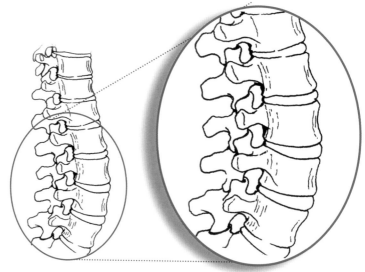

This arrangement allows for flexion, extension, and lateral flexion, but it also forms a bony "stopper" that impedes rotation.

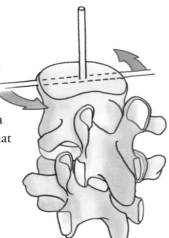

Even though a t-shirt may appear to have spiral-shaped folds in this location, torsion movement does not (or nearly does not) exist at the lumbar level.

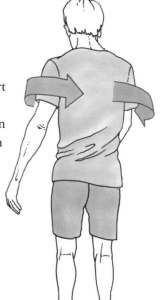

Torsion is quite easy in the dorsal spine, particularly the lower part. If we now look at the vertebral region just above (the dorsal or thoracic vertebrae), you will see that at the back, the shape of the joints has changed:

the surfaces do not block torsion at all; in fact, they favor it, by apparently being made to rotate around the intervertebral discs.

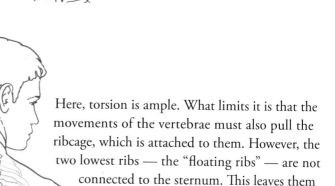

Here, torsion is ample. What limits it is that the movements of the vertebrae must also pull the ribcage, which is attached to them. However, the two lowest ribs — the "floating ribs" — are not connected to the sternum. This leaves them mobile.

From the bottom, the first place that can twist is the joint between the eleventh and twelfth thoracic vertebrae.

This is located at the bottom of the ribcage. Here, a section that is very mobile in rotation follows a section without mobility. When you force torsion, the hyper-mobile section risks becoming too mobilized, which can be the case in *Marichiasana.*

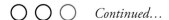 *Continued...*

It is therefore important not to "let go" of the T11 vertebra; do not let it rotate too much. It is even necessary to *restrain its rotational movement.*

This is primarily done by *a muscular action that rotates in the opposite direction*, including the deep back muscles situated closest to the spine, called the *multifidus muscles* (AOM, p. 74).

To really feel this action, here are three exercises that can prepare you.

1. Rotate the trunk from the deep muscles of the spine: sit on the edge of a chair, and feel the ischia press against the seat. Let the arms rest alongside the trunk.

Rotate your trunk and return to normal again, several times. Explore how to initiate this torsion in various ways, from your arms, your shoulders, or your ribs.

Then feel how *the spinal rotation can come from the spine itself:* the muscles that do this are deep, situated behind the vertebrae.

HALT THE ROTATION: start again, and stop the movement cleanly: these same muscles work on both sides to *secure your spine*.

2. Find L3, then T11: put your hands "on your hips," that is to say on your iliac crests. Join your thumbs. This is the location of the third lumbar vertebra, also known as L3.

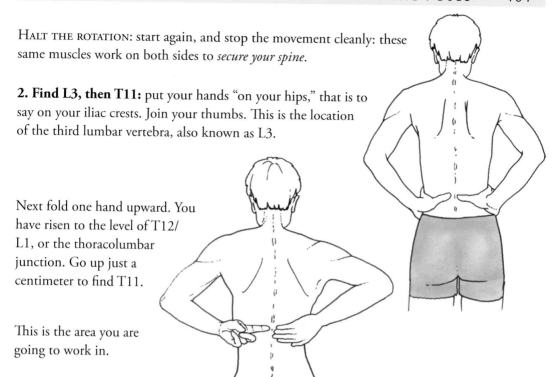

Next fold one hand upward. You have risen to the level of T12/L1, or the thoracolumbar junction. Go up just a centimeter to find T11.

This is the area you are going to work in.

HALT THE ROTATION IN ONE SECTION: with your hand, firmly rub the vertebral area at T11 several times in order to locate it well. Then repeat the rotation described above, trying to initiate the action in the area that you just rubbed. Again, stop the movement cleanly, by acting in one segment (localized static contraction). Feel how you can maintain a fixedness in this segment while continuing to breathe.

3. Actively keep a section in passive torsion: pivot on the chair, and sit to one side so that your back is about ten inches from your right arm. Cross your left arm in front of you and take the back of the chair in your left hand.

While pulling yourself, rotate the trunk towards the right: the torsion is no longer active, but passive.

Come back again. Repeat, while slowly developing the movement. As described above, try to stop the torsion at T11, as if you have *immobilized the spine at the bottom of the ribs*. Don't be afraid to start over, as this action is unusual.

● ● ●   Practice at the End

Coordinate the quadriceps and the gluteus maximus in
Virabhadrasana I (Warrior I)

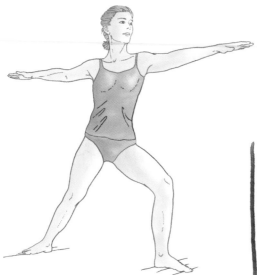

Among other things, this pose requires you to support yourself on a leg with the knee flexed. The weight of the trunk, the head, and the arms rests for the most part on this leg, whose knee must be "held" so that it stays in position and does not bend further.

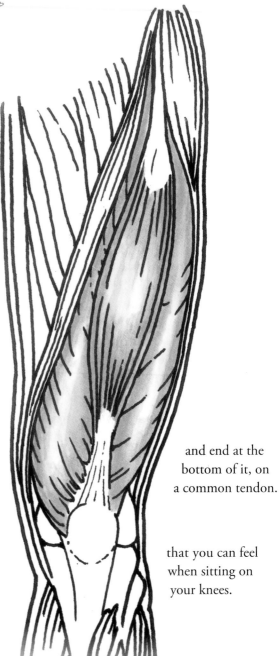

This engages the *quadriceps* (AOM, p. 238), the largest muscle of the body, formed by four parts (or "heads") that run along the front of the thigh…

and end at the bottom of it, on a common tendon.

This large tendon crosses the knee and then ends at the top of the tibia, on a well-marked bump…

that you can feel when sitting on your knees.

During flexion and extension the tendon, bent at the knee, receives considerable friction and pressure. That is why it is lined with a skeletal reinforcement, the patella. The action of this muscle is therefore inseparable from the patella, which is almost "crimped" in its tendon.

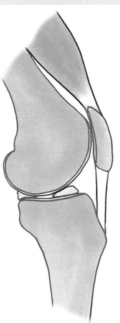

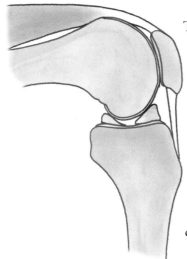

The deep face of this small bone, covered with cartilage, glides against the femur, also lined with cartilage. It supports the pressure instead of the tendon,

and for them to be balanced, it is important that the patella remain centered in the middle of the knee during movement.

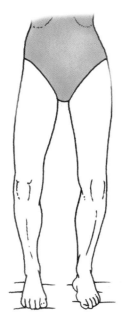

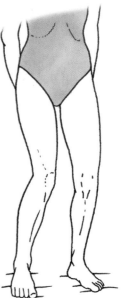

However, the leg bones are frequently not aligned correctly with one another when supporting yourself on a bent leg, and the knee, between the hip and the ankle, can be found placed a little like a zigzag.

This alignment is detrimental to the patella and to the correct placement of the foot, which has to balance itself between these internal and external supports.

Adjusting this alignment is thus a good exercise to practice before taking *Virabhadrasana I*.

○ ○ ○   *Continued…*

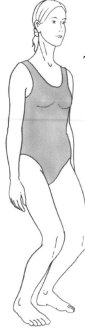

Train yourself with a simple exercise that flexes both knees: first try by keeping your feet parallel.

Bend your legs just a little, until the moment when you feel the heels begin to rise from the ground.

Do not go too far. Look at each knee: how are they placed over the feet?

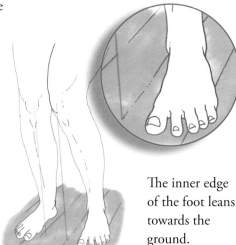

The inner edge of the foot leans towards the ground.

The knee is above the inside of the foot: your patella is poorly centered, and is pushed outward. Only slightly, but this is enough for your quadricep to engage its external head, and for the pressure to be stronger on this side. This unnecessarily strains the cartilage in the area.

Rebalance: to correct this tendency, first try to over-correct and orient the knee above the outside of your foot.

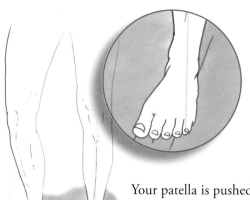

But here again, the foot is not well-placed: it is now the outer edge that rotates towards the ground and its internal supports are no longer in contact with the ground.

Your patella is pushed towards the inside of the knee (this is less harmful than the preceding case). For this correction, you have oriented the thigh and the knee a little towards the outside, an action that can be carried out by the muscle of the buttocks: the gluteus maximus. You can feel it contract in the back of the buttock.

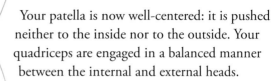

Try to place the knee vertical to the foot: now aim for above the second toe: that is where the *longitudinal axis of the foot* passes.

Your patella is now well-centered: it is pushed neither to the inside nor to the outside. Your quadriceps are engaged in a balanced manner between the internal and external heads.

The foot is well-placed: its internal and external supports are allocated evenly.

Here too, this action can be carried out by the gluteus maximus. But you can feel that its contraction is less strong.

Thus, the strength of the gluteus maximus's contraction adjusts the orientation of the femur, which allows for good alignment of the leg bones (other muscular co-ordination is possible, but is not discussed here).

Next try to rotate your feet a little, into a V towards the outside (like the front foot in *Virabhadrasana I*). This position comes from your hip, which creates external rotation.

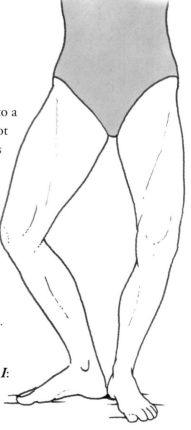

Note: The balance found in a parallel-feet position is often lost in external rotation. In this new position, try to place the knee above the second toe, without leaning to the inside or correcting too much and leaning to the outside. You will find the measured action of the gluteus maximus.

Finally, try to establish this alignment in *Virabhadrasana I*: the alignment work is now just on one leg, the leg that is flexed.

Measure the action of the quadriceps and protect the patella in *Virabhadrasana I* and *II* (Warrior I and II)

For this pose, whether variation I or II, we settle on two feet. There may be significant differences depending on whether we support ourselves more or less on one or the other. Here we will again observe the patella of the bent leg in relation to the angle of action in the quadriceps.

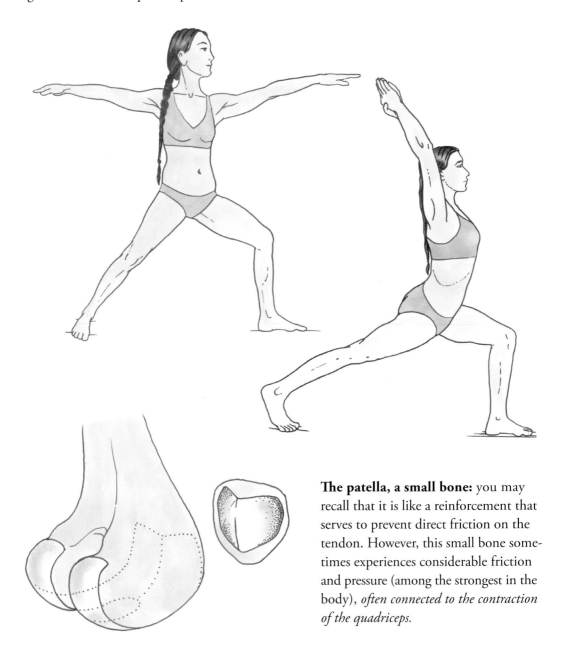

The patella, a small bone: you may recall that it is like a reinforcement that serves to prevent direct friction on the tendon. However, this small bone sometimes experiences considerable friction and pressure (among the strongest in the body), *often connected to the contraction of the quadriceps.*

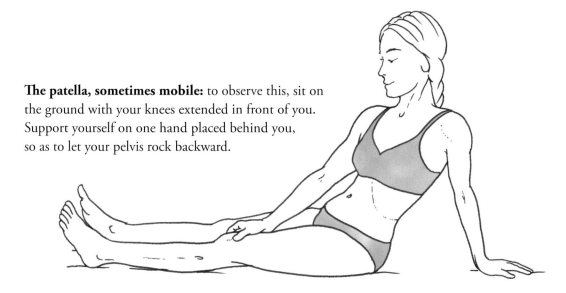

The patella, sometimes mobile: to observe this, sit on the ground with your knees extended in front of you. Support yourself on one hand placed behind you, so as to let your pelvis rock backward.

Place the other hand on the front of the knee: you can move the patella by slowly sliding it (a little) towards the inside or outside of the knee. This tiny movement indicates that the bone here is free to move a little, since the quadriceps are relaxed at this moment.

The patella is thus free and, above all, *it is not compressed.*

The patella, sometimes the site of great pressure: stand with the knees slightly bent. If you place a hand on one patella, you will no longer be able to make it glide. Its movement, though tiny, is impeded. In this position the patella is no longer free to move, since the quadriceps are contracted to stabilize your knees.

Important: it is thus strongly pressed against the femur, which can cause significant compression.

Most people can withstand this compression quite well, since the cartilage there is thick. But it creates a problem for any fragile knee: *it would therefore be better to arrange the poses systematically to reduce the pressure on the patella.*

○ ○ ○   *Continued...*

Right angle for the bent leg in *Virabhadrasana I*.
Here we can find an instruction that is always
present when practicing this pose:

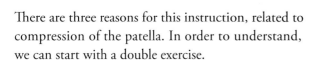

*do not bend the
knee beyond a
right angle.*

There are three reasons for this instruction, related to
compression of the patella. In order to understand,
we can start with a double exercise.

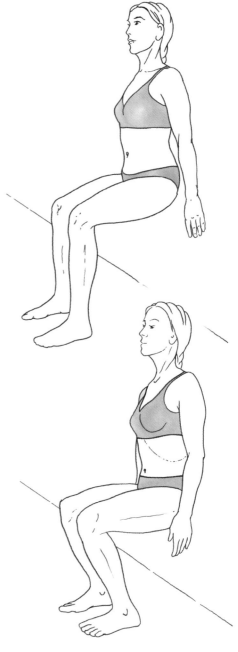

**Press your back against a wall and bend your
knees 90 degrees.** Your tibiae are vertical.

Stay there for a few seconds: you will feel the
quadriceps contract in the front of the thigh. It
prevents your knee from bending further. It acts
on the vertical tibia, *which is naturally stable as a
result of this verticality,* like a well-balanced pole.

Move your feet a little closer to the wall. Your
knees then *flex more than 90 degrees. Your tibiae
are no longer vertical.*

You are still engaging the quadriceps. But you
must also now straighten your tibiae, which naturally tend to fall forward. The contraction is
stronger ... and the compression of the patella
is stronger too. Therefore, placing the tibia vertically helps to put less pressure on the patella.

Exceeding a right angle: extra tension.
There is another reason to prefer a right
angle in the bent supporting leg. It is
that the more flexed the knee is...

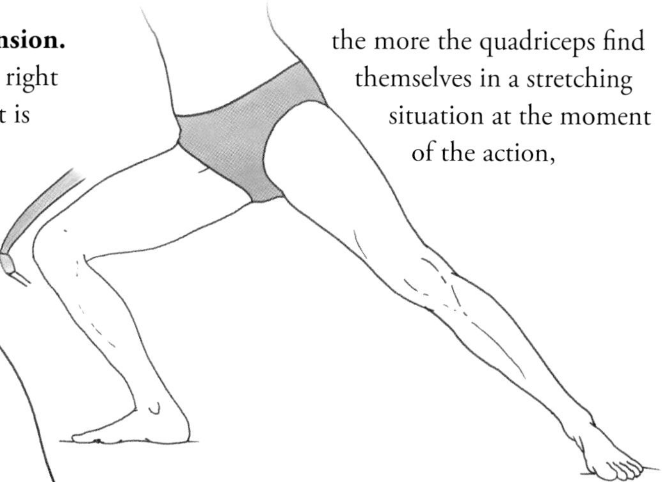

the more the quadriceps find
themselves in a stretching
situation at the moment
of the action,

compared with
when the knee
is at a right
angle.

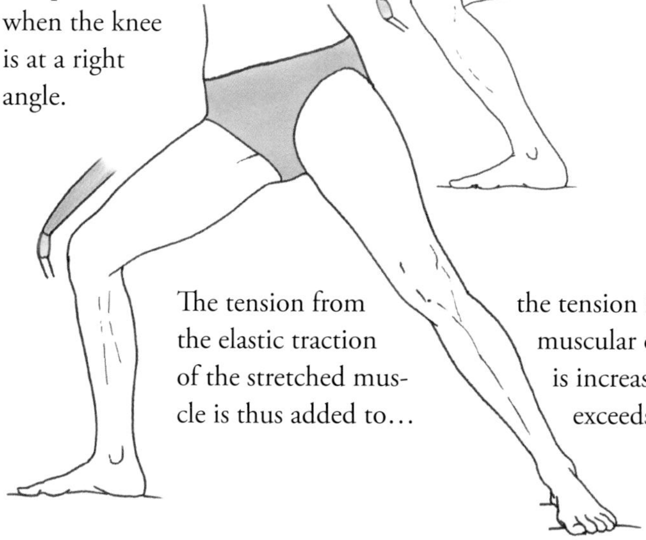

The tension from
the elastic traction
of the stretched mus-
cle is thus added to...

the tension in the tendon generated by the
muscular contraction. Here too the result
is increased compression if the flexion
exceeds 90 degrees.

**Support yourself on both feet
to relieve the bent leg.** Why do
we sometimes bend the knee
beyond a right angle?
This happens when we
carry the weight of the
trunk too much on the
bent leg, or rather...

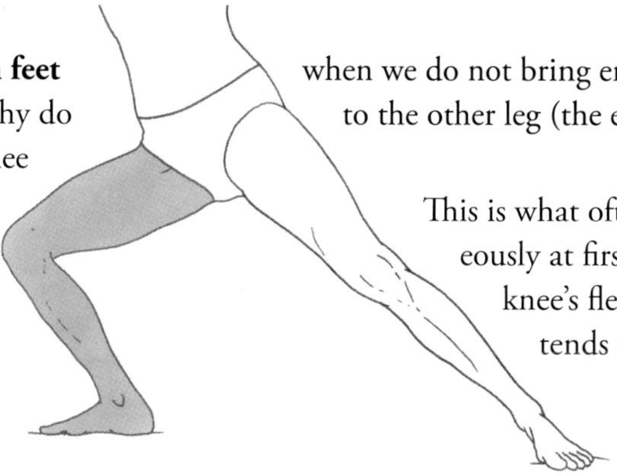

when we do not bring enough of the weight
to the other leg (the extended one).

This is what often happens spontan-
eously at first. But in this case, the
knee's flexion almost always
tends to increase.

It is therefore necessary to try to support yourself with both feet.

In order to do this, before bending
you must search for the proper
distance between the feet that
allows you to easily distribute
support onto both. This is
personal.

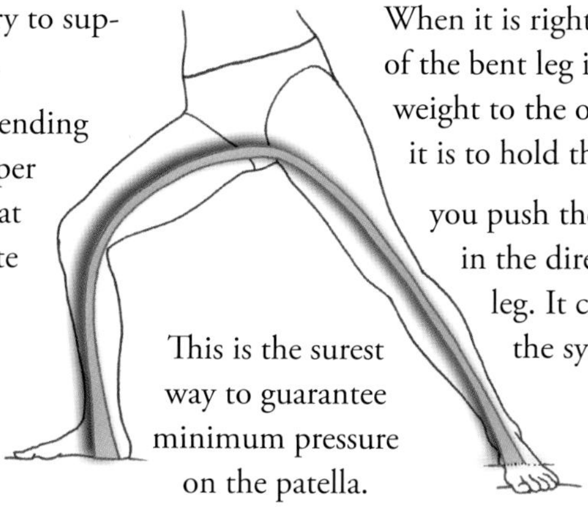

When it is right, it feels like the work
of the bent leg is primarily to send the
weight to the other leg, more than
it is to hold the bend of the knee:

you push the weight of the trunk
in the direction of the extended
leg. It creates a force that uses
the synergy of both legs.

This is the surest
way to guarantee
minimum pressure
on the patella.

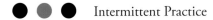 Intermittent Practice

Balance the heel in *Garudasana* (Eagle Pose) and *Vrikshasana* (Tree Pose) using the lateral ankle muscles

The heel bone, called the *calcaneus*, is an important area to understand. Sometimes it can be important to know how to "navigate" it laterally under the ankle. Sometimes, however, it is necessary to *stabilize it laterally*, in particular for *regulating balance* in the *standing asanas*, such as *Garudasana* and *Vrikshasana*.

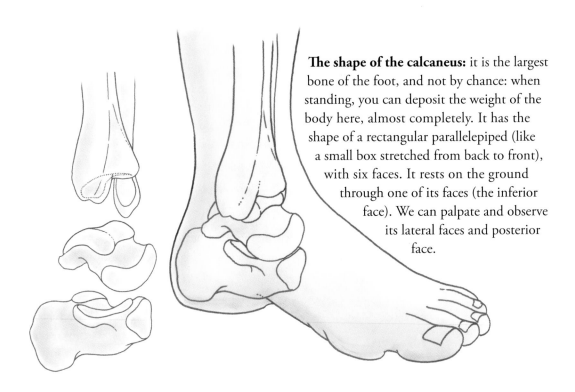

The shape of the calcaneus: it is the largest bone of the foot, and not by chance: when standing, you can deposit the weight of the body here, almost completely. It has the shape of a rectangular parallelepiped (like a small box stretched from back to front), with six faces. It rests on the ground through one of its faces (the inferior face). We can palpate and observe its lateral faces and posterior face.

Observation of the heel and the back in support: it is easiest to watch another person. But if necessary you can watch yourself from behind in a mirror. Stand on both feet. Observe the shape of the back of the heel.

Seen from behind, the calcaneus has a shape that is more or less a vertical oval. The base of the oval, slightly flattened, rests on the ground. The top of the oval is extended by the *Achilles tendon*, which continues in the calf as the triceps surae. The ensemble looks a bit like an hourglass (see the drawing on the following page).

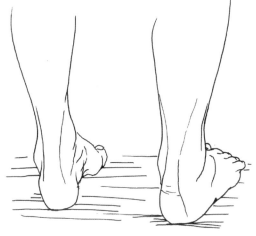

Try two possible placements first: the oval can be oblique, as if the bone "goes down" a little, on the internal side. We call this a calcaneus in *pronation*.

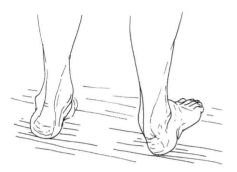

The oval can be oblique, as if the bone "goes down" a little, on the external side. We call this a calcaneus in *supination*.

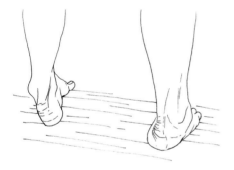

In these two cases, the Achilles tendon does not extend the oval, but rather forms an angle with it. The heel appears deflected. This has consequences for the rest of the foot, in the front, but also for the bones situated above.

The "middle of the heel": find it, leave it, and return to it. Now try to balance the foot so as to rest it in the middle of the heel, as if you were on an ice skate and you wanted the blade of the skate to be vertical.

To feel this, place a pencil under your foot, that runs along this median and leaves a sensation in the skin of the foot. Next, "load" the foot: bring your weight onto it more or less completely, while retaining the sensation and memory of the median.

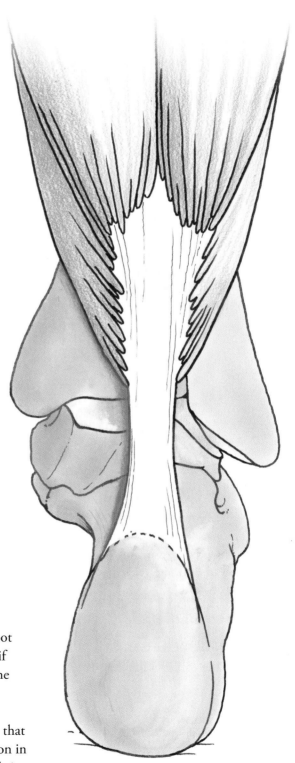

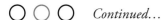 *Continued…*

In *Garudasana* (Eagle Pose). Next, go into a position of pronation: your heels lean inward. Then try to return to the "middle" position. To achieve this, you can feel the action of the muscles that pass through the internal side of the hindfoot, under the malleolus.

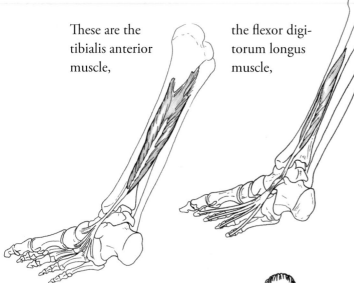

These are the tibialis anterior muscle,

the flexor digitorum longus muscle,

and the flexor hallucis longus muscle (AOM, p 290).

If you assume ***Garudasana* (Eagle Pose)** (standing on your right foot),* do you feel how the crossing of your left arm around the right tends to cause pronation in your supporting foot?

You can thus look for the precise muscular actions that pull the foot into supination.

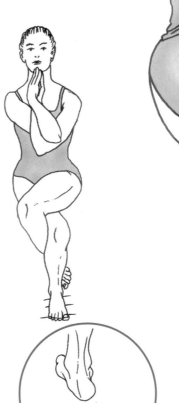

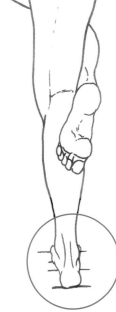

*The action is described for the right foot as the supporting foot, but the pose can of course be practiced on the other foot as well.

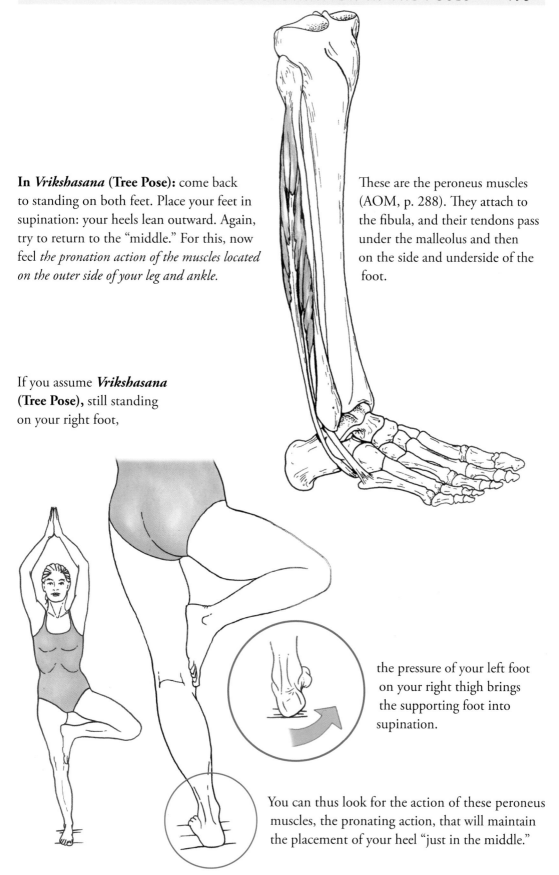

In *Vrikshasana* (**Tree Pose**): come back to standing on both feet. Place your feet in supination: your heels lean outward. Again, try to return to the "middle." For this, now feel *the pronation action of the muscles located on the outer side of your leg and ankle.*

These are the peroneus muscles (AOM, p. 288). They attach to the fibula, and their tendons pass under the malleolus and then on the side and underside of the foot.

If you assume *Vrikshasana* (**Tree Pose**), still standing on your right foot,

the pressure of your left foot on your right thigh brings the supporting foot into supination.

You can thus look for the action of these peroneus muscles, the pronating action, that will maintain the placement of your heel "just in the middle."

Contract the triceps surae to protect the knee ligaments in *Trikonasana* (Triangle Pose)

This pose places the spine in lateral flexion/torsion/ flexion, with a large offset of the trunk.

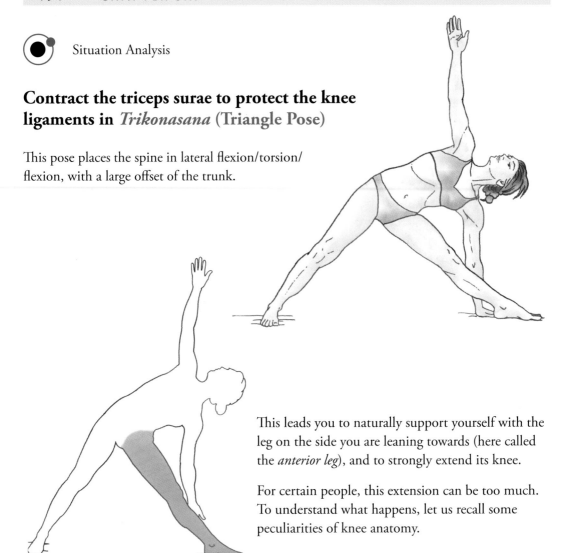

This leads you to naturally support yourself with the leg on the side you are leaning towards (here called the *anterior leg*), and to strongly extend its knee.

For certain people, this extension can be too much. To understand what happens, let us recall some peculiarities of knee anatomy.

This joint connects the two longest bones in the body: the femur and the tibia, which while standing must remain one on top of the other, securely balanced. The knee is stabilized by a capsule and some ligaments.

But it also creates very ample movements: flexion that can reach 175 degrees, and the return to rectilinear femur-tibia alignment, called *extension*. This requires the ability to mobilize the capsule and ligaments while maintaining the stability seen above.

The capsule and the tibial condyles: the capsule is a thick, fibrous sheath (like a knee pad) that surrounds the joint, with folds that enable its movements. It is very thick at the back, forming the "tibial condyles" that strongly reinforce it.

These are tensioned when the knee passes into extension, preventing the movement from going farther. They are the principal constraint to hyperextension of the knee.

The cruciate ligaments: in the center of the joint, these ligaments are arranged almost vertically, their directions partially intersecting.

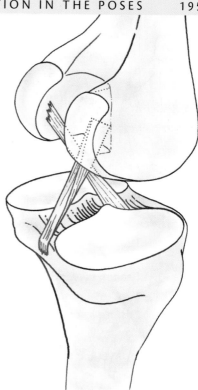

The main function of the anterior cruciate ligament (ACL) is to prevent the tibia from gliding forward under the femur.

The posterior cruciate ligament (PCL) prevents the tibia from sliding backward under the femur. Because of these ligaments, these long bones never slip over or under each other. Their integrity is vital, especially for support and for the strong and fast actions of the knee.

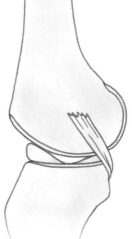

Hyperextension of the knee: in extension, the cruciate ligaments are placed in tension ("normal" tension that stops the movement). But this sometimes goes farther, creating hyperextension, which stretches them much more strongly.

Sometimes too much: they can then be stretched and weakened (the ligament, which is not very elastic, does not have to be stretched much for it to constitute a sprain).

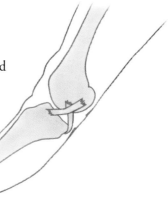

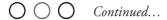

○ ○ ○   *Continued...*

Knee hyperextension: in *Trikonasana*, the weight of the trunk is shifted towards the anterior leg, which tends to increase the extension of the knee. Generally this is retained well by the tibial condyles. Certain people, however, have *hypermobility* and can extend their knees beyond rectilinear alignment. This is knee hyperextension. In a standing position, you can then observe a reentrant angle at the front. The back of the joint (the popliteal fossa), usually hollow, instead bulges outward.

Knee hyperextension is due to excessive flexibility in the tibial condyles. Hyper-extension of the knee is thus no longer prevented. *The cruciate ligaments are at risk of distention.* This is why *you must never increase hyperextension beyond its natural range.* Because of this, *it is best not to create or accentuate passive hyperextension of the knee in people who already have hyperextension.*

For these people, *Trikonasana* requires special attention: they must "hold" their knee.

Leaning on your leg in *Trikonasana*: considering the significant offset of the trunk, in the fully-developed pose it is useful to support yourself on the lower hand (so as not to overwork the disks and intervertebral ligaments).

Sometimes we place this hand on the ground, which means going down quite low with the trunk.

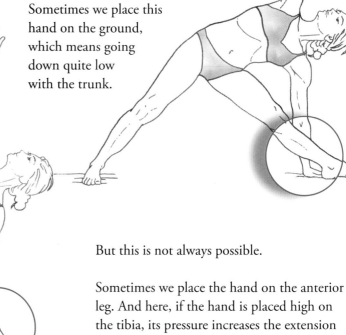

But this is not always possible.

Sometimes we place the hand on the anterior leg. And here, if the hand is placed high on the tibia, its pressure increases the extension of the knee. In light of what was said above, this type of support is not recommended for people with hyperextension.

Here are several suggestions and modifications to deal with this problem:

Support yourself with other things: you can place a support under the supporting hand (such as a firm block) to support the weight of the trunk while not leaning so far.

Keep some weight on the posterior leg: try to keep a part of the weight on the posterior leg. This relieves the anterior knee, and reduces the tendency to hyperextend.

Support yourself on an active knee: you can resist hyperextension by contracting the muscle flexors of the knee: particularly the calf muscles. For this, place a support under the front of the foot (a wedge, folded fabric, etc.), and try to press on it.

Later, you can recreate this action without the support. The sensation must be one of "keeping the back of the knee active," so that it is not drawn into hyperextension.

Note: this action should remain moderate and should not lead to tension of the entire leg.

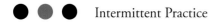 Intermittent Practice

Choose between two muscles for positioning the pelvis in
Setu Bandha (Bridge Pose **or** Half-Wheel Pose)

In this pose, the higher you lift yourself, the more the pelvis — raised above the ground — searches for its position. Here we will focus on two muscles (in reality double right-left muscles) that can orient it, with very different sensations and effects.

In a fully-developed **Setu Bandha,** you are balanced and supported on the feet and the scapulae: between these supports, the posterior parts of the trunk and the legs are above the ground.

To achieve this, you must shorten (through contraction) all the posterior parts.

The movement can begin with a push of the legs or by pressing through the arms or scapulae.

But in every case, *the pelvis tends to flex when it arrives at the top.*

Therefore, you must try to go in the opposite direction, that is to say, the direction of extension.

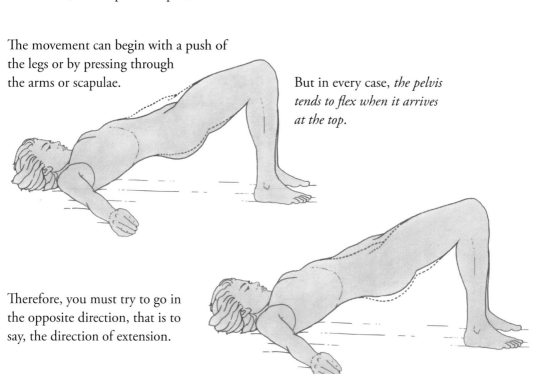

We will begin with some reminders about flexion and extension of the pelvis. These have already been introduced in the context of stretching the hamstrings for **Dandasana** (Boat Pose) (see p. 104), but they are discussed here in a totally different context.

Mobilize the pelvis and the waist: we can begin by looking at these pelvic movements in an easy and free situation. Lie on the ground, the knees and hips bent, feet flat (we will call this the *starting position*). Optional: place a soft cushion under your pelvis to mobilize it without the ground stopping it too quickly.

Feel the somewhat curved form of your sacrum, and roll it slowly in the direction of the feet, leaning towards the coccyx. This movement (flexion of the pelvis in a supine position) causes the waist region to be hollowed out, which is called *lordosis*.

Next go into the reverse movement (extension of the pelvis). The lordosis disappears in the lumbar region, and this area spreads to the ground. You can feel this by placing a hand under your waist.

Repeat these two movements. You can initiate each of them with the waist as well as with the pelvis: for example, if you hollow the waist your pelvis will be carried towards the coccyx. But you can also bring the coccyx to the ground, which will hollow out your waist.

Pelvic extension, two ways: now only go into extension of the pelvis (when the waist is in contact with the ground) and experiment with two ways to practice it, using two different muscle groups. For this, return to the starting position.

1) Push a little (just slightly) on the feet and right away find strength in the buttocks to move your pelvis. These muscles roll the pelvis by mobilizing it from behind; then, if you go farther, they raise it.

Try to only act with these muscles, even if at the start other actions are combined with that of the buttocks.

2) Still in the starting position, place your fingers on your stomach a little below the navel. Next, raise the head (just a little). Under your fingers, feel the contraction of the abdominal muscles in the front of your abdomen (the rectus abdominis muscle). Place the head back on the ground.

Now, with the rectus abdominis, try to pull the front of your pelvis in the direction of your navel: this puts it in extension, but very differently from the previous way, through work that engages your abdomen and that leaves your buttocks relaxed. The rectus abdominis mobilizes your pelvis in the front, while the gluteus maximus mobilizes it from behind.

○ ○ ○   *Continued…*

Now practice **Setu Bandha** and feel how you can make one muscle
or the other control the action.

The pelvis led by the buttocks in *Setu Bandha*: if you
contract the buttocks to lift yourself up, your abdomen
and your rib cage will be free, particularly
for breathing.

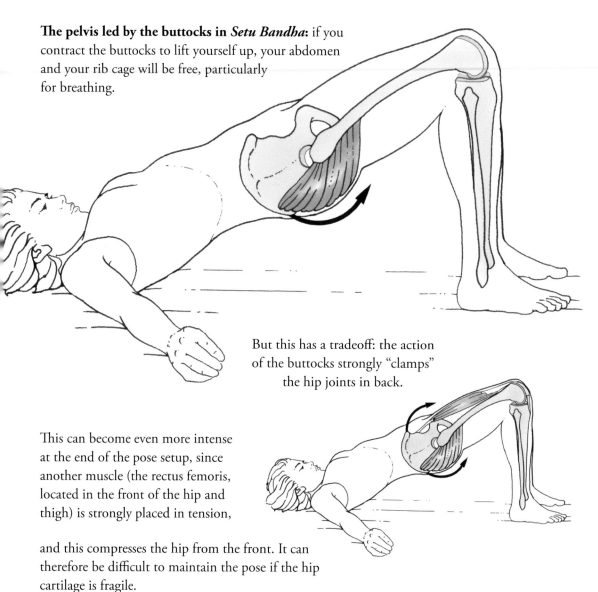

But this has a tradeoff: the action
of the buttocks strongly "clamps"
the hip joints in back.

This can become even more intense
at the end of the pose setup, since
another muscle (the rectus femoris,
located in the front of the hip and
thigh) is strongly placed in tension,

and this compresses the hip from the front. It can
therefore be difficult to maintain the pose if the hip
cartilage is fragile.

It is thus necessary to prepare well for **Setu Bandha**
by first practicing either the stretching exercises for the
rectus femoris presented on p. 126, or the poses that
lengthen the front of the hip, such as *Dhanurasana*
(Bow Pose), *Bhujangasana* **(Cobra Pose)** or
Virabhadrasana I **(Warrior I)**.

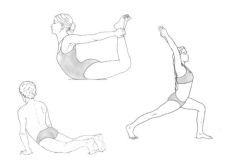

The pelvis led by the rectus abdominis muscle in *Setu Bandha*: if you contract the rectus abdominis, it is your hips that will be more free, and this is particularly advantageous if they are fragile or tired.

But it is the trunk that is now very tight in front.

Respiratory movements are momentarily impeded.

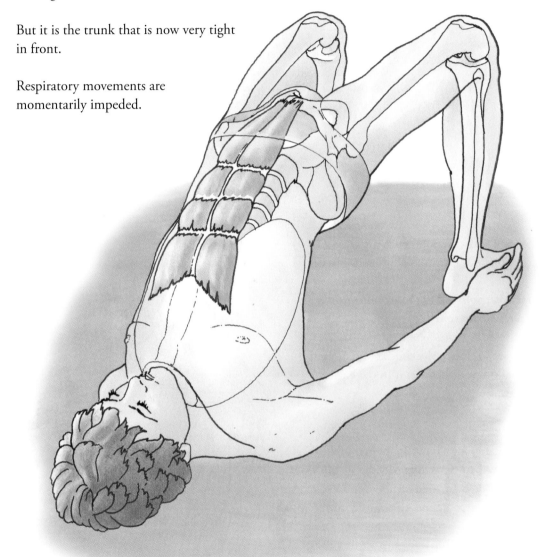

This is not particularly consequential, as this discomfort will last only as long as the pose. But it can be beneficial to prepare for it with deep breaths and with asanas that mobilize the rib cage, such as *Matsyasana* **(Fish Pose).**

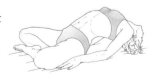

Once you have distinguished them, you can also combine these two muscular engagements so that they complement each other during the course of the pose, favoring the strength of one or the other.

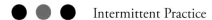

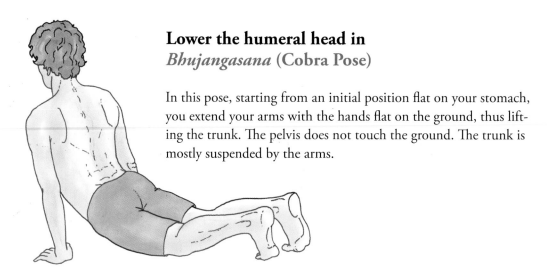

Lower the humeral head in
Bhujangasana (Cobra Pose)

In this pose, starting from an initial position flat on your stomach, you extend your arms with the hands flat on the ground, thus lifting the trunk. The pelvis does not touch the ground. The trunk is mostly suspended by the arms.

The arms must respond with a pushing action that occurs in three different places:

First area: *your elbows must maintain a powerful extension*

This may be due to the contraction of your triceps. You will then feel it in the backs of your arms.

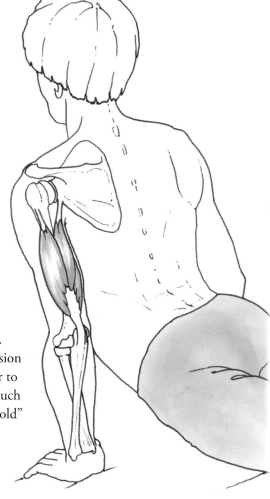

If your elbows are hypermobile, they may tend to hyperextend. In this case, it is possible for them to "wedge" bone on bone, without requiring much action in the triceps. This makes it possible to assume the pose in a less muscular way at the elbow. (However, if the hyperextension is significant, it is better to avoid increasing it. In such a case, try instead to "hold" your elbow.")

Second area: *your shoulders must stay "low"*

In fact, the weight of the trunk strongly lowers
the rib cage relative to the scapulae: feel how they
naturally tend to rise, placing "the shoulders in
the ears."

Try to respond to this gliding of the trunk by
lowering your scapulae as much as possible,
as if you wanted to raise and release your neck.
This action is carried out by your serratus anterior
(especially the lower fibers, AOM p. 120) and the
transverse region of your trapezius (AOM, p. 124),
the two muscles working in synergy-antagonism.

This gives an impression of "raising the trunk" as
much as "lowering the shoulders."

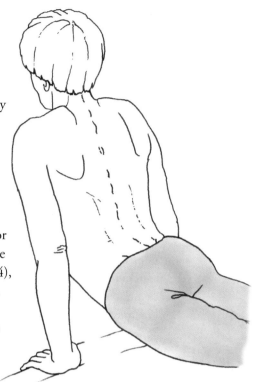

Third area: *the upper arm must stay away from your scapula*

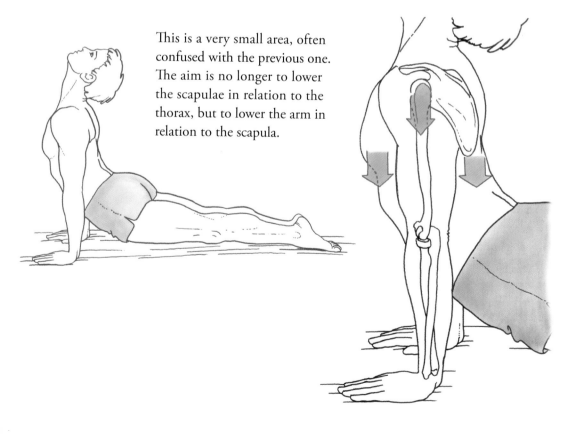

This is a very small area, often
confused with the previous one.
The aim is no longer to lower
the scapulae in relation to the
thorax, but to lower the arm in
relation to the scapula.

○ ○ ○   *Continued...*

The weight of the trunk and the head (major parts of the body) press strongly on the humerus bones. The humeral head, at the top, is at the forefront of this support dynamic. The more the trunk tends to descend, the more the humeral head is pushed upward like a piston, towards the acromion.

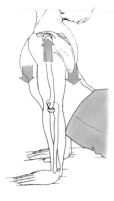

There is a place where the compression can become too significant, between the acromion, the humeral head, and the components situated between them: the supraspinatus tendon and the synovial bursa that prevent it from chafing under the acromion (these components are described on p. 82 in relation to the deltoid).

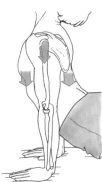

Here, it is no longer the muscle that causes the compression, but the weight of the body. Releasing the deltoid will not help.

What is needed is to actively lower the humeral head as much as possible, under the acromion.

This can be achieved through the combined action of all muscles whose actions (total or partial) draw the humerus downward:

In back:

• the teres minor, which goes from the scapula to the upper part of the humerus: this muscle is primarily an external rotator of the shoulder. But part of its action lowers the humeral head;

• the latissimus dorsi, which goes from the pelvis to the (slightly lower) upper part of the humerus: its action powerfully contributes to the descent of the humeral head.

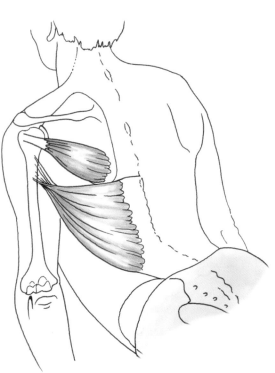

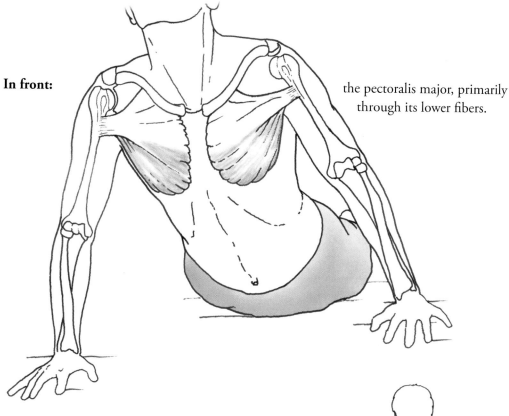

In front:

the pectoralis major, primarily through its lower fibers.

You can practice actively lowering your humerus in easier circumstances than **Bhujangasana**. For example:

• sitting at the edge of a table, place your elbow on the table so that it is almost vertical (adjust the height of the seat if necessary).

Try to push the plane of the table with your elbow. Feel the difference between lowering the scapula, and creating space between your humeral head and your acromion;

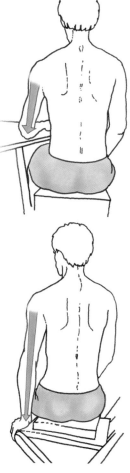

• sitting on the edge of a seat, place your hand (the part near your wrist) on the plane of the seat, also so that it is almost vertical. (But be careful, depending on the length of your arms, your hand will either reach the seat or go farther than it. Here too, you can adjust the height of your seat).

Try to push the plane of the seat with your hand. This second exercise requires extension of the elbow. Feel the difference between this extension and the active lowering of your scapula, and the active lowering of your humeral head.

Coordinate the scalene muscles for
clavicular breathing

Yoga poses often require your neck to be both supple and strong. The scalenes are among the muscles that keep the neck erect. But their action can be easily transformed.

The scalenes on the side of the neck

There are three of them on each side, arranged one behind the other (the anterior, middle, and posterior scalene) on the sides of the thin cervical spine. Important detail: they do not attach on the head.

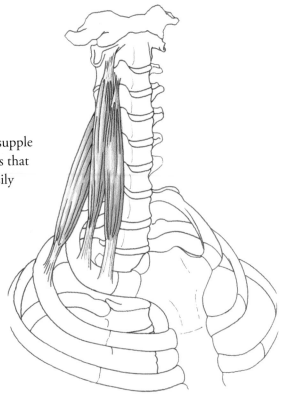

Discover the scalenes by tilting the neck to the side

Sit on the edge of a seat with your feet a little apart. Delicately place your fingers on both sides of the lower half of your neck. Do not push, but instead use light contact to feel what happens under the skin.

Then swing slowly towards the right, keeping the trunk and neck rectilinear, like a roly-poly toy. Your fingers will feel a mass harden along the left side of the neck. These are your scalenes contracting, to keep the right side of the neck from falling. You can reproduce the exercise on the left side.

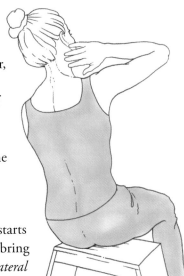

These muscles are like "stays" for the cervical spine. If the neck starts to bend to the right, they limit the movement. They could also bring it back to vertical or tilt it to the other side (left). They *control lateral neck movements*, and they work … all day long.

MUSCLE COORDINATION IN THE POSES

The scalenes as respiratory muscles: we can observe the action of the scalenes "in profile." To do so, place your left hand flat under the right clavicle. Try to inhale in a way that raises this area: here, your scalenes *have raised your first two ribs.*

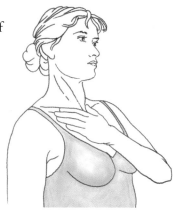

Along with the pectoralis minor, these muscles are the actors in *clavicular breathing* practiced during **Pranayama** in the "full yogic breath." But, so that they can effectively carry out this lifting of the ribs, it is necessary that…

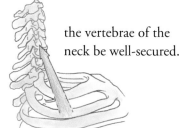 the vertebrae of the neck be well-secured.

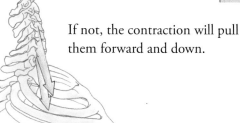 If not, the contraction will pull them forward and down.

The neck can be driven by scalenes that are too short: in some people, shortened scalenes make the neck dip towards the first rib. This is especially true when standing (*Tadasana*): the lower half of the neck is projected. The head is not above the chest, but in front of it.

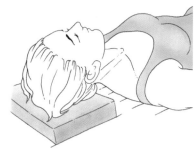

In **Shavasana,** it is difficult or impossible to place the head on the ground without a support. If they want to do so, they will find that the head tilts backwards.

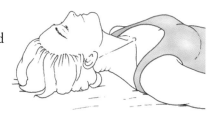

When facing this difficulty, it is useless to try to use force to realign yourself: it is better to momentarily respect this need by installing a support (a wedge) under the head, and gradually lengthening the scalenes over several weeks or months.

Two exercises can help with this.

1. Stretch the scalenes by aligning the neck on the ground: lie on your back with a wedge under the head, allowing your face to be parallel with the ground. With your hands, gently pull the head. Stay there for several minutes to allow for *passive realignment.*

2. Stretch the scalenes through torsion: slowly roll your head from one side to the other while holding it in your hands. Torsion *lengthens the scalenes.*

Appendices

General Index

A

abdominal muscles 23, 49, 51, 54, 55, 59, 152, 153, 158, 159, 175, 199, 221

abduction 21, 68, 69, 135, 150

Achille's tendon 110, 113, 190, 191

acromion 82, 83, 85, 204, 205

actin 14, 15, 100, 101

active 21, 99, 142, 169, 197, 205, 221

adductor 43, 77, 88, 90, 91, 103, 128, 129, 130, 131

adductor magnus 128, 129, 131

Adho Mukha Svanasana 18, 103, 110, 111, 214, 217

agonist 23

Anjaneyasana 29, 103, 122, 214, 217

ankle 48, 50, 51, 67, 69, 89, 108, 110, 111, 112, 113, 121, 132, 142, 144, 166, 171, 172, 183, 190, 192, 193, 220

antagonist 23, 35, 43, 166

aponeuroses 13, 16, 17, 22, 101

arch of the foot 176, 177

Ardha Chandrasana 26, 27, 77, 92, 94, 214, 217

arm 26, 42, 45, 48, 49, 51, 52, 53, 55, 57, 58, 60, 61, 62, 63, 64, 65, 74, 79, 82, 83, 84, 85, 93, 114, 116, 117, 120, 122, 137, 138, 139, 140, 141, 142, 143, 144, 145, 146, 147, 148, 149, 150, 151, 160, 161, 162, 163, 164, 165, 166, 180, 181, 182, 198, 202, 203, 205

B

back 48, 56, 57, 58, 59, 63, 67, 78, 87, 105, 108, 115, 116, 117, 118, 130, 137, 139, 140, 144, 148, 150, 160, 174, 180, 188, 190

Bakasana 47, 52, 214, 217

Balasana 77, 86, 99, 214, 217

Bhujangasana 20, 171, 200, 202, 204, 205, 214, 217

Boat Pose 43, 47, 56, 57, 59, 157, 158, 214, 217

bone 13, 14, 17, 22, 23, 39, 43, 50, 69, 82, 83, 98, 99, 110, 123, 138, 146, 150, 169, 176, 183, 185, 186, 187, 190, 191, 194, 195, 202, 220

"bony stopper" 20, 178

Bow Pose 103, 127, 142, 143, 149, 200, 214, 217

brachii (triceps brachii) 45, 64, 103, 146, 148, 166

C

Bridge Pose 45, 127, 139, 157, 166, 171, 198, 200, 214, 217

buttock 21, 72, 90, 122, 131, 137, 174, 184

calcaneus 110, 190, 191

Camel Pose 19, 29, 59, 103, 124, 214, 217

cantilever 93, 117

cap, capsule 21, 73, 146, 194

cardiac muscle 12

cartilage 183, 184, 187, 200

Cat Pose 20, 42, 55

cervical 66, 67, 87, 119, 150, 206

Chair Pose 32, 33, 47, 48, 50, 214, 217

Chakrasana 45, 157, 166, 167, 214, 217

Child's Pose 77, 86, 115, 121, 214, 217

chin 67, 87, 119

clavicle 118, 120, 138, 139, 160, 207

Cobra Pose 20, 53, 171, 200, 202, 204, 205, 214, 217

collagen 16, 17, 22, 101

compression 21, 75, 187, 188, 189, 204

concave 31, 92, 93, 95

concentric 24, 25, 26, 33

contraction 12, 14, 17, 18, 20, 22, 24, 25, 26, 27, 28, 30, 31, 32, 33, 34, 36, 37, 39, 40, 42, 48, 49, 55, 56, 59, 61, 64, 66, 67, 69, 71, 73, 74, 75, 78, 79, 80, 85, 90, 99, 100, 143, 153, 164, 169, 170, 174, 175, 176, 181, 184, 185, 186, 188, 189, 198, 199, 202, 207

convex 31, 92, 94

coordination 168, 169, 185

coracoid 140

Corpse Pose 71, 77, 78, 80, 207, 214, 217

Cow Face Pose 99, 103, 146, 148, 214, 217

Crescent Lunge on the Knee 51, 65, 103, 122–123, 139, 214, 217

Crescent Moon Pose 65, 214, 217

Crow Pose 47, 52, 214, 217

cruciate ligaments 195, 196

curving, bending 28, 92

English-Sanskrit Index of the Poses Discussed

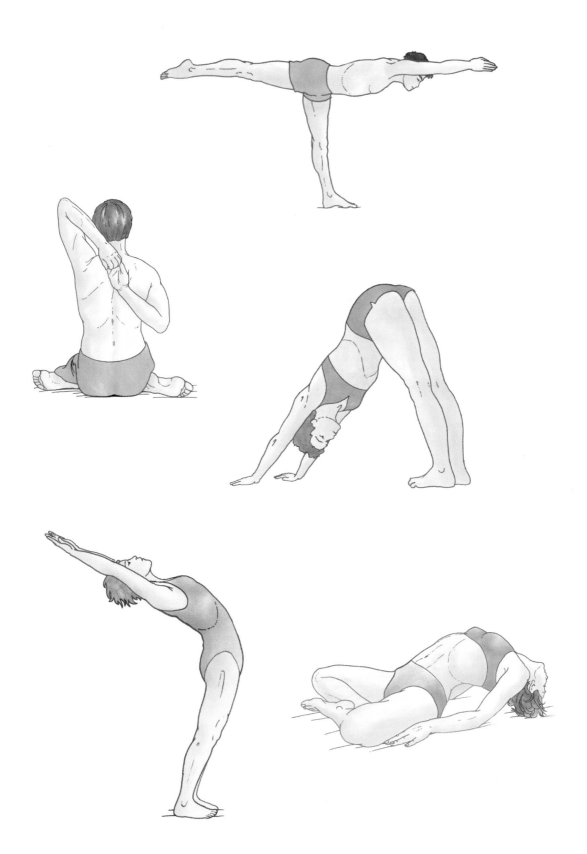

Sanskrit-English Index of the Poses Discussed

Adho Mukha Svanasana	Downward-Facing Dog Pose	110
Anjaneyasana	Crescent Lunge on the Knee	122
Ardha Chandrasana	Half-Moon Pose	92
Balasana	Child's Pose	86
Bakasana	Crow Pose	52
Bhujangasana	Cobra Pose	202
Chakrasana	Wheel Pose	166
Dhanurasana	Bow Pose	142
Dandasana	Staff Pose	104
Garudasana	Eagle Pose	150
Gomukhasana	Cow Face Pose	146
Halasana	Plough Pose	188
Hasta Uttanasana	Raised Arms Pose	138
Kumbhakasana	Plank Pose	58
Malasana	Garland Pose	114
Marichiasana	Seated Spinal Twist	178
Matsyasana	Fish Pose	62
Natarajasana	Lord of the Dance Pose	162
Navasana	Boat Pose	56
Paschimottanasana	Seated Forward Bend	116
Padmasana	Lotus Pose	132
Purvottanasana	Upward Plank Pose	58
Salabhasana	Locust Pose	60
Samakonasana	Straight Angle Pose	128
Sarvangasana	Shoulderstand	152
Shavasana	Corpse Pose	78
Setu Bandha	Bridge Pose/Half-Wheel Pose	198
Sirsasana	Headstand	66
Supta Baddha Konasana	Supine Bound Angle Pose	88
Tadasana	Mountain Pose	172
Trikonasana	Triangle Pose	194
Utkatasana	Chair Pose	48-50
Ustrasana	Camel Pose	124
Vrikshasana	Tree Pose	68
Virabhadrasana I	Warrior I	182-186
Virabhadrasana II	Warrior II	186
Virabhadrasana III	Warrior III	164

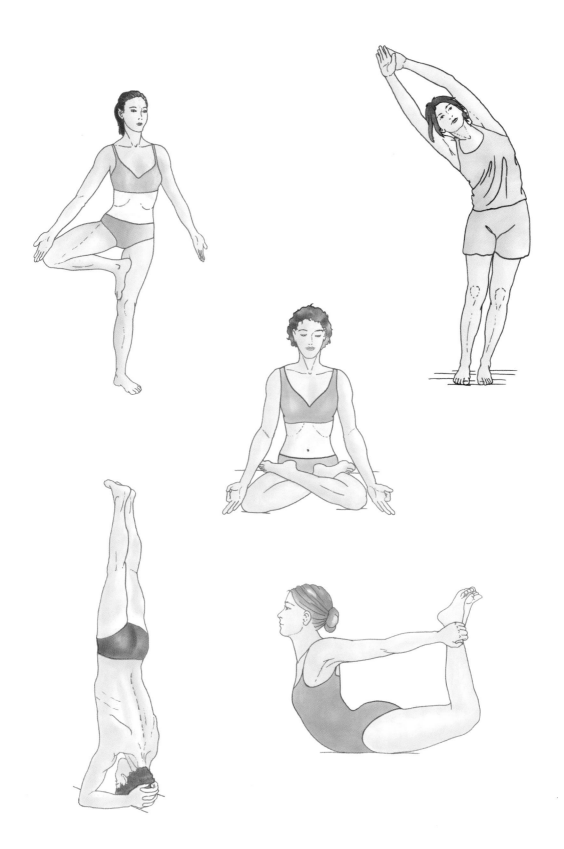

Bibliography

A. Bouchet – J. Cuilleret
Anatomie topographique, descriptive et fonctionnelle, Simep, 1990

C. D. Clemente
Anatomy, Urban & Schwarzenberg

F. Netter
Atlas d'anatomie humaine, Masson, 2005

Gray's
Anatomie pour les étudiants, Elsevier Masson

J. Brizon – J. Castaing
Les feuillets d'anatomie, Malonie

W. Kahle, H. Leonhard, W. Platze
Anatomie, Flammarion

H. David Coulter
Anatomy of Hatha Yoga, Body and Breath

N. Perez Cristiaens
Attention le Yoga peut être dangereux pour vous, ISA

L. Kaminoff
Yoga: anatomie et mouvements, Vigot

R. Long
Yoga anatomie, Les muscles, la Plage

B. de Gasquet
Yoga sans dégâts, Marabout